Treatment of Depression in Managed Care

Mental Health Practice Under Managed Care
A Brunner/Mazel Book Series

S. Richard Sauber, Ph.D., Series Editor

The Brunner/Mazel Mental Health Practice Under Managed Care Series addresses the major developments and changes resulting from the introduction of managed care. Volumes in the series will enable mental health professionals to provide effective therapy to their patients while conducting and maintaining a successful practice.

Mental Health Practice Under Managed Care, Volume 7

Treatment of Depression in Managed Care

Mark Mays, Ph.D., J.D.
and
James W. Croake, Ph.D., ABPP

Brunner/Mazel, *Publishers* • New York

Library of Congress Cataloging-in-Publication Data

Mays, Mark.
    Treatment of depression in managed care / Mark Mays and James W.
Croake.
    p. cm. – (Mental health practice under managed care ; v. 7)
    Includes bibliographical references and indexes.
    ISBN 0-87630-829-9 (pbk.)
    1. Depression, Mental–Treatment. 2. Managed care plans (Medical
care)   I. Croake, James W.   II. Title.   III. Series: Mental health practice
under managed care ; 7.
    [DNLM: 1. Depression–therapy. 2. Depression–diagnosis. 3. Depressive
Disorders–therapy. 4. Depressive Disorder–diagnosis. 5. Managed Care
Programs–United States. W1 ME9268 v.7 1997 / WM
171 M474t 1997]
RC537.M3924   1997
616.85'27–dc20
DNLM/DLC
for Library of Congress   96-36748
                                                                            CIP

Published by
BRUNNER/MAZEL, INC.
19 Union Square West
New York, New York 10003

Manufactured in the United States of America

10   9   8   7   6   5   4   3   2   1

To my family, and those friends who are like family.
They keep my life full and fun.

Mark Mays

To Dr. Harold Mosak, my mentor and guide
over the past 30 years.

James W. Croake

Contents

Preface

This is a book designed for mental health practitioners, with a secondary audience of mental health plan administrators and other policy makers in the mental health arena. We discuss the managed care context as it affects treatment for a common mental health problem–depression. We approach this subject from slightly different perspectives, with a variety of experiences in mental health delivery. Together we have provided psychological services through Native American projects, military health care systems, academic clinics, private practices, free clinic volunteer activities, and health maintenance organizations, as well as managed care organizations. The settings were hospital based and nonhospital based, including continuous inpatient and outpatient treatment and consultation.

The primary author, Mark Mays, Ph.D., J.D., developed and administered one of the first federally funded health maintenance organizations in the 1970s–the Cooperative Health Plan. In private practice for the last two decades, he has also served on a state licensing board in psychology and held state and national offices in psychology. Mays is also an attorney, and he draws upon a training approach which encourages apprizing matters from a variety of perspectives. James Croake, Ph.D., ABPP, has had a breadth of experience in academic settings. He has served as a preceptor in the training of psychiatric residents and postgraduate psychology students in both outpatient and inpatient settings, and he has consulted to mental health clinics, hospitals, and family medicine clinics and

ix

published extensively, with an emphasis in marriage and family therapy. We share a focus on individuals as existing within a social context. We enjoy a systems perspective, which considers the influence of forces and factors external to the individual important in treatment.

From these backgrounds and this perspective we approach the task of mental health delivery on a practical level. Although the book starts by discussing the context of managed care, forms of brief therapy, and ways to understand, measure, and conceptualize depression, our primary concern is how to treat depression. We believe that understanding and deliberateness precede effective action, certainly in treatment, and, we hope, in the approach taken in this book. The keys to managed care will almost certainly be treatment planning, outcome assessment, quality control, and practice standards. Knowledge of syndromes and methods of assessment, as well as of tools and techniques, will be vital on the practical level of therapeutic intervention.

Managed care is a moving target, one that is quickly changing. Certain trends do seem apparent, even though it is hard to predict the exact form they might take. We hope that we have gauged these trends correctly, and that the information that we have synthesized and presented is relevant to providers treating patients in practical and meaningful ways.

Acknowledgments

Over the years, I've always skipped over the acknowledgments in books and considered them somewhat unimportant. Having spent the last months in preparing this book, I realize how many people are vital to its completion.

Sally Garves and Renee Stamps provided helpful transcription services for the initial drafts. The secretarial staff at Dr. Croake's office provided transcription assistance in the complex task of editing the initial drafts. As the work became more technical and exceeded their time availability, I was fortunate to have discovered Jan Hansen, without whom this book literally would not have been completed. Jan provided knowledge and flexibility, precision and dedication. She helped in bibliographical documentation and attempted to ensure that citations were accurate through the many drafts. It is one thing to have a coauthor whom you believe to be brighter and more knowledgeable than you. One is doubly blessed to have a transcriptionist of similar abilities.

One of my concerns through all of this has been that the work of others would be misquoted or perhaps not sufficiently acknowledged through the various revisions. I was concerned about this not only out of a commitment to editorial convention, but also out of a great and growing appreciation and respect for the significant work done by some giants in the field upon whom I have relied. I wanted to ensure that they were acknowledged for their work and contributions, which provided the foundation upon which this book is built.

My good friend Ron Klein, Ph.D., provided editorial comment throughout the revisions. His quiet and scholarly manner were much appreciated. How he can maintain such a serene and gentle nature in today's world is a mystery to us all. Michael Freeman, M.D., President of the Institute for Behavioral Healthcare, provided time, support, encouragement, and advice. Richard Sauber, Ph.D. has been a source of information, guidance, and support throughout this project.

Natalie Gilman at Brunner/Mazel was always pleasant, supportive, and flexible. I come from a family with many involved in publication fields and know that delays are never welcome. As we were delayed in completion through misfortunes of health and unexpected complexities, Natalie was always kind and supportive. Suzi Tucker and her staff added editorial skills and much of their valuable time in refining the presentation of our work. Thanks!

Finally, and most of all, I thank my family for their patience and good nature while this project took my time and attention.

MARK MAYS, PH.D., J.D.

My thoughts are echoed in Dr. Mays's comments with regard to the breadth of helpfulness that we have received and the continuous concern for accuracy and representation in our citations. Richard Sauber has once again shown his skills in the most helpful manner.

I would like to also acknowledge the help and support of P. P. LaBarge, R. Staub, J. Block, and especially Durive.

JAMES W. CROAKE, PH.D., ABPP

1

Managed Care

Managed care is the new environment in which mental health care is being delivered. In biology, environments determine which species flourish and thrive, and which species dwindle and decline. Harsh environmental changes may cause some species to disappear altogether, as has the dinosaur, and as might the snail darter. Ecological environments nurture and support certain species, but not others. Some species thrive on what an environment provides, and others cannot adapt to the sustenance available. Survival is a dance between the environment and the organism, where compatibility defines survival.

This applies to health care as well. Managed care has become the environment and determines the ecology for the delivery of health care services. Some "species" of mental health care will flourish, and others will fade. As an environment, managed care supports those approaches which focus on change, value efficiency, define goals, allow flexibility of treatment approach, and achieve measurable results. Theories and therapies in mental health which support those treatment approaches will grow. Other therapies are less concerned with measurable results and embrace more subjective and intrapsychic changes. Some therapies propose treatment approaches which may take years as they strive to explore character restructuring and the modification of global patterns of personal organization in the context of a slowly evolving therapeutic relationship. Perhaps sadly, these theories will not be compatible with the new health care milieu and will not gain the reimbursement necessary to continue.

1

The community of mental health professionals has been attentive to the changes that are occurring with the increased involvement with managed care. Articles discuss "coping" with managed care. Focus groups, such as that conducted in 1994 by the American Psychological Association (APA, 1994), show concerns and complaints about managed care which "cut across all focus groups." As was noted, "almost universally, the participants expressed regret about what they believe will be the ultimate impact of managed care on their patients and themselves." Managed care is seen by many, particularly those with a psychoanalytical point of view, in themes reminiscent of mourning. Others see the changes as oppressive and compare managed care to a "totalitarian regime" (Shore, 1995). Fox (1995) discusses the "rape of psychotherapy." Others employ a metaphor of war and write about "battling" with managed care. The old way of doing things seems to be on its last legs, and a sense of loss, fear, and anger characterizes the mood of the provider community.

It also seems quite clear that managed care is here, and here to stay. Managed care membership has increased. Up to 90% of those Americans receiving mental health care benefits will receive these services through managed care organizations or arrangements by the year 2000 (Freeman, 1995). In its 1992 survey, *Psychotherapy Finances* found that 66% of interviewed therapists had already signed managed care contracts. Be they Health Maintenance Organizations (HMOs), Preferred Provider Organizations (PPOs), Employee Assistance Programs (EAPs), Competitive Medical Plans (CMPs), Independent Practice Associations (IPAs), or "carve-out plans" such as those administered by Greenspring or U. S. Behavioral Health, such organizations, acronyms, and arrangements will continue to be the context of mental health delivery in the future.

These changes will have profound effects on the mental health professions. Cummings (1986), long recognizing the proliferation of mental health costs and therapists, discussed the trends accompanying these excesses many years ago. Actuarial predictions of efficient utilization, such as that achieved in managed care, indicate the need for perhaps one qualified therapist for every 5,000 people. This would create the need for approximately 50,000 psychiatrists, psychologists, social workers, and mental health counselors for the

250 million people in the United States. At present there are approximately 250,000 such therapists licensed and certified in the United States, a ratio of about 1 per 1,000 people. Many predict that up to 50% of all currently practicing psychotherapists will be out of business by the year 2000 (e.g., Cummings, 1988; Freeman, 1995). There are those who see the fee-for-service private-pay arena that has characterized mental health for the past 30 years as passing away. They are not just imagining its death.

WHY MANAGED CARE?

Managed care is a solution to a problem, and the problem it is attempting to solve is real. Some health care costs have increased by two to three times the national inflation rate over the past 10 years (Berman, 1987). Although there are some indications that this is slowing, the trend is still alarming. Particularly when costs of health care in the United States are compared with health care costs in other countries, the trend is a cause for concern. For example, in the 1980s the average annual expenditure for health care costs in the United States exceeded $1,900 per person, as compared to $500 per person in Japan and $400 per person in England (Ludwigsen and Enright, 1988). Japan spends 6.7% of its Gross National Product (GNP) on health care, with outcome measures comparable to those of the United States. At present, health care costs in the United States exceed 12% of the GNP and are projected to escalate to well over 15% of the GNP by the year 2000 (Davies and Felder, 1990). If costs continue to rise at the current rate, health care costs could consume the entire GNP of the United States by the early decades of the next century. Cummings (1995a) notes that all 250 million Americans could receive health care in 38 megaorganizations the size and efficiency of the Kaiser Permanente HMO, but requiring only 290,000 physicians (half the number in practice today) and at a cost of only 5% of the GNP.

Mental health care costs have also increased. In one year alone, corporate giant GTE's outpatient costs for mental health increased 46%. Mental health costs have increased to over 15% of the total health care budget. The number of mental health therapists has also increased radically. The largest group of treating therapists are at the Master's level. This group has grown to constitute a population of over 130,000 currently licensed in counseling or social work. New graduates are being produced at the rate of over 5,000 per year from over 500 programs. Not only are there more therapists than in years gone by, but more people are seeing therapists. Session lengths have increased, and the cost per visit has risen in the private-pay world. Utilization has increased far beyond what would be expected by assessment of risk or epidemiological studies. There is no question but that something needs to changed.

Managed care is a response to these issues by policy makers, patients, and purchasers of health care resources who are concerned about cost, access, and the quality of those services. It is an attempt to reduce health care costs by using resources in a deliberate way while simultaneously ensuring access to and quality of care. Managed care today takes several forms. Health Maintenance Organizations, or HMOs, are the oldest example of managed care structures, dating back to the early 1900s with the formation of the precursors to still operating plans such as Kaiser Permanente in California and Group Health in Washington. DeLeon, VandenBos, and Bulatao (1991) observe that until the 1980s the terms "managed care" and "HMO" could be used interchangeably. Today these plans offer a range of outpatient and inpatient medical and mental health services to an enrolled population for a per-person amount settled in advance, known as a "capitated rate."

Many other forms of managed care followed in the 1980s. Preferred Provider Organizations, or PPOs, were formed to offer financial incentives to consumers who select a limited group of "preferred" providers of services at a reduced rate of reimbursement. Employee Assistance Programs (EAPs) for acutely distressed workers and Competitive Medical Plans (CMPs) for Medicare beneficiaries also evolved and provided limited mental health services. Other structures exist, and many others will develop, but all will attempt to use management concepts of control and deliberate use of limited resources.

The scope of managed mental health care has increased due to traditional fee-for-service private-pay insurance plans adopting managed care programs. In contrast with the old fee-for-service reimbursement arrangements, managed care today has a variety of manifestations. The "first generation" of managed care networks in mental health were "carved out" of the benefits packages of insurance companies and administered separately by managed care organizations or companies. These intermediary managed care companies would ensure that treatment was in fact necessary and authorize services to providers who had been reviewed and credentialed. Treatment was often authorized for a fixed number of sessions, and preauthorization for services was required. Utilization review, credentialing, and monitoring of patient satisfaction were frequently functions of these organizations. This gatekeeper and monitoring role evoked much protest from the provider community. The American Psychological Association member focus groups revealed a number of concerns about confidentiality, limitation of treatment judged necessary, and review by managed care staff who were seen as less knowledgeable than the provider to make health care decisions.

Carve-out systems still exist, but there has emerged a second generation system known as "provider care organizations," a form of practice association with the capability of contracting for care. These groups may have a number of different disciplines in a linked practice, and they may conduct provider monitoring and quality assurance activities internally. They may even contract with managed care organizations, health maintenance organizations, or other groups. These organizations have taken a number of forms, and it can only be assumed that they will continue to evolve. In fact, a very strong argument can be made that the next few years will see only "transitional" delivery systems, which may bear a faint resemblance to later and more effective forms of medical and mental health delivery. Many, such as Cummings (1995b), predict the ultimate demise of carve-out systems. Various forms of managed care will almost certainly unfold to target economic goals through various practice structures, but care will almost certainly be managed.

The future of health care is very hard to predict, and the exact form that managed care will take will probably be determined by the creativity of therapists, researchers, and managers; interpretations of other public policy issues which might be reflected in laws and regulations, such as antitrust law; studies persuasive to purchasers of health care or insurance companies regarding the cost savings of providing mental health care; and other such variables, including chance. Although the specific form or manifestation of managed care is hard to predict, however, one can make some reasonable predictions for *trends* that will likely be reflected in whatever organizational structures unfold.

Mental health care is likely to be increasingly delivered in an organized health care marketplace by provider groups, often integrated with medical care (Drum, 1995). There is likely to be an increasing emphasis on capitation, which is the reimbursing of groups for providing mental health services on a cost-per-capita basis. Capitated systems do not reimburse providers for units of treatment which are delivered in response to a mental health problem. Instead, groups of providers are paid a fixed amount for each member of that patient population, whether they require care or not. The provider group is then charged with the responsibility of providing care, regardless of utilization. Capitated systems tend to limit costs to the purchasers of health care insurance, and many see them as vehicles for increasing the creativity of the providers of such services. Capitated systems are seen as rewarding providers for efficient delivery of services, in contrast to unregulated reimbursement for services provided, which is thought to reward inefficiency.

Contracts for service delivery will almost certainly be with organizations, such as provider groups, and not with individual providers. A patient will turn to an organization for care rather than being referred to an individual provider. That organization will have the responsibility for providing the appropriate level and duration of care. Care may involve the use of specialists for such interventions as medication, psychotherapy, health education, or family treatment. It is quite conceivable that half a dozen providers could respond to an individual's personal and family problems, particularly if these problems compromise medical functioning. Treatment will be team treatment, on both the contract and the delivery level. It should be kept in mind, however, that the managed care provider group members will need to be linked through communication and information networks, not necessarily by physical proximity.

Quality assurance efforts will be a vital component of managed care efforts. Quality assurance programs are essential, particularly with capitated systems, which might reward providers for maintaining rates of utilization which are lower than necessary and appropriate. Provider evaluations may address patient satisfaction, rate of therapeutic success, utilization rates, and peer assessments. Less sophisticated programs may assess such things as number of rings until a phone is answered and the giving of directions to an office, all easy to measure but of questionable relevance.

NOT ALL OF THIS IS BAD NEWS

Not all of these changes are necessarily "bad news." While there has been much provider distress, there has been no indication that managed care lowers the quality of care provided. In fact, if accessibility to care is considered one of the criteria of effective health care, managed care can help resolve the dilemma of inaccessibility to care for those tens of millions currently unable to receive *any* mental health care. It has also been argued that with the escalating cost of care, access to conventional care would be increasingly limited on an economic rather than a rational basis.

Purchasers of managed health care programs have been happy with the results. Surveys assessing the effectiveness of managed care show cost savings (Curtiss, 1989). Compulsory utilization review has been found to reduce the rate of hospitalization, length of stay once admitted, and overall medical costs (Burton, Hoy, Bonin, and Gladstone, 1989). The ratio of cost savings for such managed care efforts is also high. Feldstein, Wickizer, and Wheeler (1988) found that for every dollar spent on cost containment, there was an $8 savings in overall medical costs. The proportion of administrative costs of health care is far greater in the United States than in other countries, in some cases by as much as twice as high (Woolhandler and Himmelstein, 1991), but few complain about these administrative programs, which bring about an eight-to-one level of savings.

Although quality of care is hard to measure, satisfaction with care is not. Studies show great satisfaction with managed care programs. A majority of both union and corporate leaders surveyed found that the majority detected no change in quality, only about one in eight thought it to have declined, and more than a quarter thought quality had improved (Alvine, 1989). While some studies evaluate satisfaction with overall health care and do not focus or select out mental health care, most patients and purchasers seem content with the overall changes which are taking place in health care delivery.

Although the mood in the provider community seems grim, some note an opportunity with this amount of change. Nicholas Cummings (1995a) views this as a time of "golden opportunity" for those with creativity and energy. There are other bright spots from the provider's point of view, chief among them that *mental* health services are now included in most health care policies and most proposals for health care reform. Mental health care is acknowledged to serve not only the needs of the individual patient, but also to further other societal goals.

One of the benefits of effective provision of mental health care is the reduction in costs on the primary medical care level. *Many* studies have shown that appropriately provided outpatient mental health services reduce the utilization of more expensive medical and surgical services. This results in an overall decrease in health care expenditures (e.g., Hankin, Kessler, and Goldberg, 1983; Borus and Olendzki, 1985). These findings have been reported for a number of populations: high medical utilizers who are not experiencing life-threatening illnesses, medical patients with severe illness, patients diagnosed with a major mental disorder, and entire populations receiving health care benefits which include mental health coverage. Many believe that this cost offset is sufficiently great that mental health care, in effect, pays for itself.

The "Hawaii Medicaid" project (Cummings, Dorken, Pallak, and Henke, 1990) targeted high medical utilizers with a program designed to help them solve life problems and build social support, using psychotherapy as way to coordinate these efforts. Compared to a matched control group, those receiving these services reduced medical utilization by over $4 million. Similarly, Tulkin, Frank, Bernstein, Aubel, and Lehn (1992) found that a chronic pain program produced a reduction in medical utilization of over 40%. Although these studies are not conclusive, they do point to hopeful possibilities for justifying expanded outpatient mental health services aimed at populations of high medical utilizers.

Perhaps a different way to view the same population, or phenomenon, is to examine the medical utilization rates of those with diagnosed psychological disorders. Katon, Ries, and Kleinman (1984), in a study of primary care patients, found that 18% scored in the moderate-to-severe range for depression on two different rating scales. Follow-up studies showed that this group made more than twice the number of medical visits, called more often, and received more diagnostic testing than nondepressed cohorts. Katon observed that not all depressed patients were high medical utilizers, however. Some who were depressed never returned after the initial visit. Those who did return used the services *very* extensively. In another study, Katon and Sullivan (1990) demonstrated that over half of medical high utilizers in a large sample scored well into the clinical range on a screening test of psychiatric symptoms. Almost three quarters of the high utilizers had symptoms suggestive of a somatization disorder. Kessler, Steinwachs, and Hankin (1982) demonstrated that those receiving psychiatric care also reduced medical utilization significantly, with effects continuing for up to two years after completion of psychiatric intervention. Eisenberg (1992), writing in *The New England Journal of Medicine,* concludes that "between 11–36% of all general care physician visits involved patients with diagnosable psychiatric disorders."

The studies show that even those with serious physical illness can realize cost savings in their medical care with the addition of mental health services. Belar (1991) showed that offering mental health services to those with medical conditions such as diabetes, hypertension, and even cardiac disease results in improved morbidity rates, reduced hospital readmission rates, and better medical compliance than for those not receiving mental health benefits. Lechnyr (1992) found these medical cost savings to be as high as 18 to 31%.

Research also shows that more than 70% of the cost of mental health services goes to inpatient services (e.g., Ackley, 1993). Studies have demonstrated that provision of outpatient services can dramatically reduce the risk of more expensive hospitalization with no increase in patient risk. Mays (1979) found that offering outpatient services in a very accessible way reduced inpatient utilization to less than 25% of that predicted by actuarial studies. CHAMPUS

increased its outpatient costs from $81 million to $103 million between 1989 and 1990, but reduced inpatient utilization as a result to
the point of achieving a net gain of $200 million in overall cost
reductions (*Psychiatric Times,* August 1993).

Estimates of potential savings from accessible and effective mental health care are dramatic. The National Institutes of Mental Health
(NIMH) released a study (Goodwin and Moskowitz, 1993) which
found that providing reimbursement for mental health care to the
same degree as for medical care would cost $6.5 billion, but result
in a savings of $8.7 billion. These estimates do not even take into
account the nonmedical costs to society for mental and emotional
disorders. Kamlet (1990) estimates that in 1990 major depression
accounted for more than $20 billion in lost workdays alone. Jansen
(1986) claimed that 80 to 90% of all industrial accidents were ultimately attributable to the direct or indirect effects of psychological
or substance-use problems. Patients suffering from major depression were one and one half times more likely to be unemployed or
on welfare than nondepressed patients, and those with panic disorders were three times more at risk for such vocational deficits than
nonanxious cohorts (Markowitz, Weissman, Oullette, Lish, and
Klerman, 1989). Stress accounts for 10% of industrial disability
claims. It has been reasonably estimated (Rice, Kelman, Miller, and
Dunmeyer, 1990) that in 1985 mental illness and substance abuse
resulted in $77.2 billion in lost income. The costs of untreated psy-
chological and psychiatric disorders is staggering if one looks at
all of the economic effects.

Mental health services require mental health practitioners for effective and cost-effective treatment. Currently about 50% of all
mental health care is provided on the primary medical care level
and not by mental health specialists (Narrow, Regier, and Rae, 1993).
Beardsley, Gardocki, Larson, and Hidalgo (1988) found that more
than two thirds of all psychotropic medications are prescribed by
general medical practitioners. Research in the costs and benefits of
providing mental health care on the primary medical level indicates this is not cost-effective nor likely to be responsive to the depth
of patient needs. Coyne, Schwenk, and Fechner-Bates (1995) found
that family physicians detected only 3% of patients who met the
criteria for major depression as diagnosed on the Center of Epide-

miological Studies Depression Scale (CES-D) supplemented by structured clinical interviews. However, they did detect and treat almost three fourths (73%) of those with depressions so severe that they interfered with a patient's capacity to work. In an extensive study, Sturm and Wells (1995) found that treatment of depression by GPs following usual practice guidelines is not cost-effective. Katon (1995), writing in *JAMA*, finds that depression can be treated on the primary care level, but most effectively in a multimodal program which emphasizes education, medicines, monitoring by psychiatrists, and frequent medical visits at the start of the program—even if not medically necessitated.

These findings indicate that there will be much justification not only for mental health services to be provided, but for them to be effective. Eliminating mental health benefits or imposing utilization constraints which preclude effectiveness seems very shortsighted and is unlikely to persist. The sociologist Vilfredo Pareto proposed that society tends to reinforce the optimum use of its resources. Reducing the costs of mental health outpatient care by merely limiting access, and thus increasing costs in other parts of the medical system or reducing productivity in the workplace, would seem ill-advised, a view also held by Ackley (1993). If the health care system encourages system-wide cost reductions, as might occur in a single payer system, utilization of mental health benefits might even be encouraged.

Paul Eckert (1994) reaches similar conclusions from the perspective of quality control. He holds that short-term expenditure reduction, if at the cost of reducing quality, is less effective than the pursuit of maximal value, which he defines as the level of quality yielding the greatest possible degree of long-term cost containment. He relies on William Deming's (1986) view of the "customer's" needs as determining the nature of services an organization provides. He proposes that Deming's view, widely held in the health care arena, is better understood if the term "customer" is substituted for "recipient, beneficiary, or client," and that, throughout society, the needs of the person receiving services should determine the priorities of the person providing them. Although acknowledging that there may be more than one "customer," such as the employer and other societal beneficiaries, Eckert is clear that more than merely economic relationships are involved in health care. He advocates that a synthesis of quality and costs be the goal of managed care. Taking a broad perspective, Eckert concludes with the optimistic view that "[t]he essence of a solution lies in recognizing that there may be no fundamental conflict between improving quality and containing costs. In the final analysis, continuous quality improvement may actually be the only reliable path to long-term cost control."

It is clear from the closer scrutiny of delivery of mental health services that there are valuable cultural benefits to be gained by treating psychiatric and psychological conditions. The conditions have to be treated in ways that are demonstrably effective, and delivery has to be provided in an efficient health care system. While it is quite likely that economic forces will shift the historic expectations of the relationship between patient and provider, reduce patient choice somewhat and provider autonomy substantially, there will be much need for treatment. It is even likely that mental health services will be more available than before the managed care era. Still, chance and politics may complicate policy and access. Rashi Fein, Harvard medical economist, is quoted as saying that "in health care the invisible hand is all thumbs" (in Stone, 1995). Knowledge of relevant research on the part of the clinician in contact with policy makers, combined with future research efforts, might serve to make the "invisible hand" of the marketplace a bit more adept.

This view of the context within which managed care has evolved and exists indicates that managed care is more than merely abbreviated treatment. Managed care is different from traditional care in nature as well as in duration. It is a different way of conceptualizing both patients and the task of therapy. It not only manages providers and health care resources, it also implies the management of patient symptoms so as to decrease their presence. Managed care will likely demand that the focus be upon treating syndromes, problems, skill deficits, or other such symptoms that may exist in populations of patients, rather than on providing services to self-referred individual patients in one-to-one therapy. Goals will be defined and focused, implied not only by diagnosis but also articulated in a treatment plan, which specifies and may behaviorally define an outcome. Goals will also be measurable in order to assess task accomplishment. There will be an emphasis on practical solutions to problems which produce measurable changes, rather than on intrapsychic changes that may be assessed only by inferences from external behavior, are harder to measure, and are more subjectively based. This is an era of "getting it done" rather than a time to journey comfortably.

There will be an emphasis on the therapist managing change. There will no longer be the metaphor of the greenhouse created by the therapist, the environment for growth created by a nurturing, supportive, and well-boundaried relationship. The therapist will not watch patiently to see what insights, growth, or choices will emerge on the part of the client. It will not be a journey of discovery, but one of direction. This is a metaphor of building and constructing, rather than of growing or tending. This is an era of treatment planning and outcome assessment.

The psychotherapist in managed care might be more appropriately compared to the mechanic than to the gardener. With a mechanic, the customer's complaint defines the scope of intervention, and the "customer" may be the purchaser of health care as well as the patient. The customer whose car has slightly misaligned wheels, a malfunctioning rear power window, and a noise from the alternator, might come to the mechanic's shop concerned about none of these problems, but wanting the ignition fixed since the car occasionally won't start. The mechanic would be confined to answering the consumer's request. A helpful mechanic might notify the owner of other problems that could use attention, including repairs the customer could do unassisted, but it would be surprising for a mechanic to intervene uninvited beyond the specific request for repairs. In fact, consumer protection laws often prohibit such surprises.

The analogy of the mechanic does not suggest that people are machines but that managed care will seek to achieve specific but often limited results by utilizing the special skills, knowledge, experience, and training that the professional brings to the relationship. Managed care focuses on getting one better, and "better" has a specific, predefined, and often delimited meaning in managed care. Treatment is designed to correct specific signs and symptoms that are so personally unacceptable to the patient or the social context in which the patient lives that a diagnosis of a mental and emotional condition is made. Treatment is not designed to help with all problems in living. Treatment is defined as reducing the presence of symptoms or reducing their occurrence. Managed care exists to deliver appropriate treatment effectively, and appropriate treatment is that which is found to be effective and potent in achieving specific results. Managed care itself evolved to achieve specific system results in the cost and quality of health care, and this creates a "trickle-down" effect in which the therapist will have to achieve specific results.

Given that there are explicit goals and the inherent demand to achieve them efficiently, the most effective therapist in this new environment will use a multitude of tools and resources to move towards therapeutic goals. The therapist will be accountable to achieve results by whatever mechanisms and resources are appropriate. The therapist may be seen as more of a "change manager" than an individual change agent. Change does not need to occur in the therapeutic session. It merely needs to occur. The therapist may administer and create treatment plans which rely upon ancillary resources, as well as provide treatment personally. The therapist is there to make sure that change is accomplished. He or she is not necessarily the person who accomplishes this change. One gets no "extra points" for therapeutic progress with occurs as a result of psychotherapy in a psychotherapeutic relationship. One only gets "credit" if therapeutic changes occur. Rule-bound procedures will be frowned upon, and practical solutions will be applauded. Payment will not be based on unit of service, but will ultimately depend on achieving goals which are defined both by the patient and by those systems which coordinate patient care and refer patients to groups of providers. The most laudable of psychotherapeutic relationships, the most exquisite of insights and understandings, and a powerful patient reexperiencing of emotionally charged events, can be a deepening and rewarding experience. It will not be applauded, rewarded, or even considered relevant to the process of managed care if it does not produce measurable progress toward specifically defined and endorsed treatment goals.

We live in a new world, one that requires new responses. These responses can be learned. Those who learn new ways to conceptualize and treat mental health problems and patients are likely to be the only ones treating them.

2

A Brief Primer on Brief Therapy

Many people confuse brief therapy and managed care. They are not the same thing. Brief psychotherapy is one of the tools that managed care may employ. A sophisticated and evolved view of managed care regards brief therapy as only one of many system components used to achieve an overall reduction in the presence of emotional disorders among a defined population. Until such sophistication is more widespread, much of managed care will be provided in "carve-out" programs with limitations on length of treatment. Individual psychotherapy, rather than more integrated and system-wide interventions, will probably be the primary tool that managed care employs in the near future since this is the structure for service delivery currently in place in the private sector.

Various therapeutic interventions are designed to achieve specific goals. If treatment is focused on the task of minimizing symptom presentation for a particular patient at a given time, brief forms of psychotherapy, or a limited trial of medicines, may be sufficient. If the goal is more broadly construed, however, as including perhaps a reduction in primary medical care utilization, one can envision a situation in which families would be encouraged, urged, and cajoled to make use of weekly treatment, regardless of symptom presence, if it maintains a family's functioning to the point that patients, such as the brittle juvenile diabetic, can avoid hospitalization. Here, longer-term therapy might be the most appropriate tool to achieve the behavioral goal of adherence to a diabetic management program. Wayne Katon (1995) has urged medical practitioners to schedule frequent visits with somatizing patients at the start of treatment, even if it is not medically necessary. So, too, might algorithms and decision trees for various treatment goals be developed that urge greater, rather than lessened, use of certain forms of treatment in order to achieve specific goals.

One example of how economic structures of delivery might affect treatment is illustrated by the varying ways a delivery system might respond to recurrent depression. Continuation of therapy is indicated to reduce the rate of the highly probable recurrences of major depressive episodes. A managed care company concerned with future or inpatient costs might encourage such continuation of therapy, just as a managed care company at risk for medical costs might encourage more extensive therapy to reduce primary medical utilization. Managed care organizations with a more limited focus might set a policy to reduce utilization in both situations if the goal is only to reduce the short-term cost of outpatient care. A thoughtful approach to utilization and therapeutic outcomes may take time to evolve, however. In the meantime, brief psychotherapy will be the kiosk with the long line of buyers in the managed care marketplace.

Brief therapy is a concept and a philosophy as much as it is specific and consensually defined. Use of the term has ranged fairly widely. Malan (1976) has discussed brief therapy as including up to 50 sessions within a year, although most view brief therapy models as constituting fewer than 20 patient visits. Some (e.g., Talley, 1992) focus on very brief therapy (VPT), discussing therapeutic interventions in the three-to-five session average range. Talmon (1990) even discusses single session therapy. This range of applications—from 1 to 50 sessions—complicates research about brief therapy. Some point to brief therapy as more than a limit on the number of sessions, but also as a philosophy about therapy which necessitates a particular therapeutic approach. Many look at the values and manner of approach, rather than merely the number of sessions, as the distinction between brief and longer-term therapy. This seems to be a meaningful distinction.

When one looks at the research on psychotherapy utilization over the past several decades, it is clear that brief therapy has been used for a long time without being explicitly named. Research outcome studies show that many people have participated in treatment for short periods, and that many do not complete the entire course of psychotherapy as it was originally conceived by the psychotherapist. Previously, many of these cases were seen as examples of attrition from treatment. Some were seen as treatment failures. Others were seen as "transference cures," in which there was symptomatic relief without a major change in underlying personality problems.

The data on utilization has been clear, however. Fiester and Rudestam (1975) reviewed studies which showed that between 37 and 45% of adult outpatients dropped out after the first or second session of treatment. Other studies revealed discontinuation rates between 21% (Littlepage, Kosloski, Schnelle, McNees, and Gendrich, 1976) and 39% (Spoerl, 1975). Talmon (1990) studied utilization rates for the health maintenance organization at the Kaiser Permamente Medical Center in Hayward, California. He found that the modal length of therapy for every one of the 30 psychiatrists, psychologists, and social workers was a single session. This means that the most frequent rate of utilization was one visit. In fact, 30% of all patients who participated in treatment came for only one session over the course of a year. When they were offered another appointment, even with a small copayment or no copayment, many chose not to keep it. Talmon later studied 100,000 scheduled outpatient appointments during the period of 1983 to 1988 and found a consistent incidence of single session use of therapy. When all of the utilization rates are taken together, the average utilization for outpatient benefits for most populations averages about six sessions per year for those who actually make use of mental health benefits.

There were many explanations for these "fallouts" from treatment. It was thought that these patients failed to receive benefit of treatment, or that they left for a reasons irrelevant to therapeutic outcome. With a rekindling of interest in brief therapy, however, many of these assumptions have been called into question. It now appears that many of the patients who have been treated briefly have been treated very effectively. The research that supported this conclusion wasn't very well acknowledged, nor did it receive much attention. For example, Kogan (1957) followed up on those who failed to keep subsequent agreed-upon appointments after a single interview. He was able to interview in person or by telephone 80% of the 141 cases so designated and to gather data from their treating therapists. He found that, whereas the therapist attributed these terminations to a lack of interest or to resistance on the part of the client, the clients indicated that "reality-based factors" such as money difficulties or transportation prevented continuance, or that the situation had improved and they saw therapy as no longer necessary. In fact, about two thirds of the clients felt that they had been helped.

Silverman and Beech (1979) did a similar follow-up study of 47 people out of a pool of 184 in a mental health center who had terminated their planned treatment unilaterally after only one visit, without it being terminated by the provider. Of the 47, 70% expressed satisfaction with services, and 79% reported that the problems that had brought them into treatment had been solved. Talmon (1990) reported a study of 200 patients selected for follow-up which found that 78% said that they got what they wanted out of a single session and felt much better.

This research leads to some interesting conclusions, the primary of which is the possible lack of a strong relationship between length of treatment and benefit from treatment. Although the data is derived from actual utilization rates and does not constitute controlled research studies comparing planned brief therapy with long-term therapy, the studies which have examined duration and effectiveness of treatment have generally not shown that lengthier and time-unlimited treatments are more effective. In fact, Luborsky, Singer, and Luborsky (1975) reviewed eight studies comparing time-unlimited treatment with time-limited treatment. Of these, five showed no difference, one showed time-unlimited treatment to be more effective, but two actually favored time-limited treatment.

It would be wrong to conclude from this that all therapy can cease after one or two sessions with similar effectiveness as with that currently being provided with an average length of therapy of six sessions. It is very likely that those who could benefit from shorter-term treatment do so and exit, leaving many of those who persist in treatment to be those who might well benefit from longer-term interventions. A Japanese taxicab driver once said, in what may have been a misguided attempt to reassure a passenger, that there were only professional drivers in Tokyo because "the amateurs were killed off long ago." Budman and Gurman (1988) also point out that some of the articles comparing "brief therapy" with "time-unlimited therapy" may make very mistaken conclusions regarding their comparative effectiveness, since some of the naturalistic studies average six sessions while some brief-therapy studies may actually involve more sessions. In effect, the "brief therapy" may last longer than time-unlimited therapy in some of the research studies.

If anything, this data and its possible misuse almost requires that the mental health professions take a careful research look at therapy utilization and point out the implications for quality control to the managed care organizations. We believe there is much wisdom in Paul Eckert's (1994) article (cited in Chapter 1) that advocates a value on cost control through quality improvement—pursuing a maximum value, which is the level of quality yielding the greatest possible degree of long-term cost containment. A shortsighted and incomplete view of the utilization data could be misused, to take a fairly ludicrous example, to justify limiting all psychotherapy benefits to one session per year, based on a misinterpretation of the data that any effects, if they are to occur, occur during that session. This would be shortsighted not only for patients and therapists, but ultimately for a managed care organization which needs to develop ways to meet the very real needs of a defined population rather than to "miss the mark" through a misunderstanding of the data. Not only are many therapists new at the managed care game, so are many managed care companies, administrators, and decision makers.

Some studies show that there is something of a "stepping-stone" ranking of intervals for which different people are most likely to gain optimal improvement from therapy. For example, Howard, Kopta, Krause, and Orlinsky (1986) explored data across studies and found that between session one and session eight the percentage of patients displaying measurable improvement increased from 15 to 50%. After the 25th session, the proportion had increased to 75%, with an additional 10% receiving benefit by the end of the year. This would suggest that gains can occur early in therapy, with progressively diminishing returns over time.

Still, this may indicate that different patients benefit from different lengths of treatment. Limiting treatment arbitrarily to a fixed number of sessions without attending to the peculiar characteristics of differing Axis I conditions, particularly as complicated by Axis II syndromes or other moderator variables, might result in treatment limits which are not adequate to achieve optimal outcomes. Ackley (1993) refers to David Barlow's treatment of anxiety and panic disorder. His highly regarded research clinic specializes in treating anxiety disorders in a very focal way, but still averages eleven sessions per patient. Barlow's research (1991) indicates that seven sessions would have at best a very short-term impact and that, while medication does provide some symptom relief, the results are temporary. Examining only more immediate results, as compared to more enduring factors, necessitates redefining effectiveness of outcome and raises questions as to which standard should be used to measure "a benefit of therapy."

It is an interesting question, and the issue is far from resolved. When one explores various measures of improvement, comparing outcome studies in traditional environments to those in the more controlled environments in managed care, and adds into the equation such variables as the presence of external support networks, therapeutic style, varying definitions of therapy, client-based factors, therapist-based mediators, and contextual modifiers, much still is unknown. It is clear, however, that more is *not necessarily* better, certainly not for populations, and perhaps not for some individuals or conditions.

The data also suggest that there may be a great divergence between client measures of and therapist measures of improvement and benefit. Although therapy can be terminated by the therapist, by the patient, or by both, many of the studies explore attrition from treatment that is patient determined. For perhaps the majority of these, as suggested above, the patient often claims to have benefited and to have achieved treatment goals, but the therapist may have concluded that this is not the case. This implies different goals for treatment or very different ways to understand the goals. It might be concluded from this that therapists tend to focus on the *process* of treatment as being a goal in and of itself, while clients or patients are much more determined to seek a specific *outcome*.

There is evidence that brief therapy can help, particularly as one looks at patient indicators of outcomes and objective measures of symptom improvement and not merely at therapists' inferences derived from the data.

The possibility of iatrogenic effects of therapy, which would probably be more likely to occur in a longer course of therapy, is not often discussed. Negative effects of treatment have received short shrift in the research literature. Hadley and Strupp (1976), in a survey of researchers and practitioners in psychotherapy, found an overwhelming affirmation of the existence of occasional negative effects. Bergin (1980), Franks and Mays (1980), and others have written on the continuing debate on whether psychotherapy may in fact *cause* deterioration with some patients and whether there is research support for this. One interesting review by Terrance Campbell (1992) surveyed a year's worth of articles in a psychotherapy journal to investigate what inferences therapists might make about significant others in their clients' lives. It was found that significant others are almost always portrayed in critical ways by therapists. This raises the question whether therapists might disregard the strengths and resources of significant others in a client's life. The tendency to focus on relational problems more than relational strengths can cause iatrogenic ill effects in the social context of the client receiving longer-term treatment where the therapist's views might be more influential. As mental health therapists and researchers explore the effects of therapy, it seems that intellectual integrity and a concern with societal needs would also require some attention to be paid to possible negative outcomes with different kinds and durations of therapy for different populations.

CHARACTERISTICS OF BRIEF THERAPY

All these data, along with the economic data, have prompted a greater interest in recent years in the briefer forms of therapy. Brief therapy differs qualitatively, as well as quantitatively, from other forms of therapy. Brief therapy is usually characterized by a time-limited nature, a focus on therapeutic goals, and an emphasis on patient feedback and collaboration.

The collaborative nature of treatment and the egalitarian roles of patient and therapist seem more than justified by a variety of outcome studies. Many studies show that it is the client's view of the therapeutic process that is critical, if not predictive, of outcome (e.g., Luborsky, Crits-Christoph, Alexander, Margolis, and Cohen, 1983). Rudolph (1993), in an interesting article on midpoint review in Brief Collaborative Therapy, discusses a mechanism for incorporating the patient's views in treatment. She advocates refocusing on goals and possibly revising the therapeutic approach at the midpoint of a time-limited course of treatment. Rudolph believes the process of midpoint review allows the therapist to model the therapeutic goals of observation, self-review, and self-disclosure. She recommends facilitating communication with the therapist by focusing on four criteria for treatment: goals, tasks, the nature of the interpersonal bond, and the context of the treatment.

Brief therapy assumes a time limit at the outset (Hoyt, 1990). Several therapists see an inherent value in setting time limits to treatment. Mann (1981) notes that "time-limited psychotherapy, with its time restrictions and its particular method for selection of the central issue, cannot help but bring to the forefront of the treatment process the major pain that human beings suffer, namely the wish to be with one another but the absolute necessity to learn how to tolerate separation and loss without undue damage to one's feelings about self." Mann conceptualizes treatment from a psychoanalytic perspective, but sees a role for brevity. Otto Rank (1947) also proposed having as a therapeutic focal point the limits on time itself, this being a metaphor for other limits within which one must exist. Budman and Gurman (1988) viewed the deliberateness of time limits as vital in understanding the brief therapy process. Budman points out that the distinction in philosophy and attitude of the brief therapists is reflected in the acknowledgment that there are limited time and professional resources to accomplish a task. He distinguishes brief therapy by design from brief therapy by default (Budman & Gurman, 1988).

Brief therapy needs to be focal. Butcher and Koss (1978) believe that brief therapy of any kind must have a central issue or topic. A focus for treatment may be helpful regardless of whether treatment is brief in nature or not limited in duration. DeBerry (1987) views psychotherapy from a phenomenological framework and sees it as a "relationship with a focus." He sees both the relationship and the focus as necessary factors for the creation of a therapeutic alliance. DeBerry sees iatrogenic distortions in psychotherapy as stemming from an overemphasis or underemphasis on one of these two factors of relationship or focus. Whether the problem is defined by the therapist, as seems reflected in some psychoanalytic therapies, by the patient, or in a more collaborative way, the focus on a problem seems to differentiate brief therapy from many other forms of therapy.

Brief therapy also seems to have a *specific* problem focus. As such, it tends to focus more on the presenting problem and to seek solutions to specific problems rather than addressing the more underlying pathology and attempting "character restructuring." Brief therapy is not a "flawed personality" therapy. Klerman, Weissman, Rounsaville, and Chevron (1984) note that one of the difficulties in training experienced therapists for interpersonal therapy is their tendency to overemphasize problems as characterological and therefore have great difficulty adhering to a limited problem focus in treatment.

The brief therapist wants change to occur by whatever means are available, not necessarily to "be there" as the patient makes these significant changes. The brief therapist is quick to use a variety of resources in order to enhance, supplement, or even replace aspects of therapeutic change that might occur during the formal psychotherapy hour.

Some brief therapy models are implicitly psychosocial in their focus and mechanism. Brief therapy tends to be quite attentive to the individual existing in a specific social context, rather than merely as a person only existing within the course of the therapeutic hour.

Finally, as so well described by Walter and Peller (1992), brief therapy is also solution focused. The focus in therapy is not only upon what the problem is or what prompted it, but upon the positive outcome that a patient seeks. Brief therapy seems to focus on the patient's resources and skills and to emphasize strengths that can be built upon to achieve the solution that the patient seeks and in which the therapist concurs. The old song said, "You have to accentuate the positive, eliminate the negative." One would say that brief therapy aims to "accentuate the positive in order to eliminate the negative," with "the positive" being both the focus on the patient's strengths and the positive outcome that the patient seeks.

SCHOOLS OF BRIEF THERAPY

There are some "formal" schools of brief therapy. Budman and Gurman (1988) have developed Interpersonal Developmental Existential therapy (IDE) as a form of brief therapy, which is defined as "an attempt to capture and understand the core interpersonal life issues that are leading the patient to seek psychotherapy at a given moment in time, and to relate these issues to the patient's state of life development and to his or her existential concerns."

An implicit question in such treatment is, "Why now?" Although the IDE therapist is certainly curious about the patient's point of view, he or she does not necessarily adopt it as the "true cause." Acknowledging that patients' moods may influence their view of the past and cause them to define acute problems as more chronic than they really are, the IDE therapist would listen carefully to the patient but draw his or her own conclusions.

IDE also assumes some commonality in developmental pathways in all adults' life spans. Relying on Cohler and Boxer's 1984 book on adult development, the IDE Therapist focuses on common foci, or source points, of disruption in previously adequate levels of functioning. Developmental difficulties, interpersonal conflicts, symptomatic presentations, and certain predictable losses may be shared by many. This approach certainly opens the door to group treatments for certain common developmental issues, such as empty-nest losses for homemakers, adjustments to military retirement for middle-aged males, and the like.

Mann (1981), as noted earlier, defends a psychoanalytic form of brief therapy. Malan (1963) proposes an anxiety-provoking brief therapy with the aim of resolving a patient's central problem as interpreted by the psychoanalytically trained therapist. Sifneos (1979) is somewhat similar to Malan but with more of an interpersonal focus of concern. Sifneos uses confrontation as a way of helping the patient experience transference, and he sees resolving negative transference as one of the goals of brief therapy. Strupp and Binder (1984) have written on time-limited dynamic psychotherapy, and many other schools (e.g., Davanloo, 1980) have been developed. It should be noted that some of the briefer psychoanalytic therapies are "brief" primarily as compared to longer-term psychoanalytic therapies. Malan, for example, in proposing a time-limited focus, notes that therapy may last between "twenty and forty sessions" or "until a patient and therapist feel the matter is resolved." Many might be hard-pressed to view this as a school of brief therapy in a world in which the average trial of psychotherapy is about six sessions and social forces are attempting to reduce this number.

Klerman et al. (1984) have developed an interpersonal therapy geared towards depression. The focal point of treatment in Interpersonal Therapy (IPT) is the interpersonal themes or patterns outside of treatment and how symptoms are associated with interpersonal relationships. IPT is structured and focuses upon such common issues as grief, interpersonal disputes, role transitions, and interpersonal deficits. Klerman (1984) has developed a helpful manual for IPT which allows it to be defined and thus researched. There is evidence that IPT is as effective in certain forms of depression as compared with treatment using only tricyclic antidepressants and yields superior results in combination with them (DiMascio, et al., 1979; Weissman, 1979).

It is interesting that both amitriptyline and IPT were found more effective than control groups, but the two had different effects on symptoms. IPT improved mood, work performance, and interest, reduced suicidal ideation, and diminished guilt. The effects tended to endure throughout treatment. Amitriptyline had an effect mainly on vegatative signs of depression, such as sleep and appetite disturbance. A follow-up one year after treatment suggested that IPT, either alone or in combination with medicines, showed a better improvement in patient functioning and social activities as parents, in their families, and overall (Weissman, Klerman, Prusoff, Sholomskas, and Padian, 1981). There were no negative effects of combining IPT and medication, and the positive effects of each seemed additive. As will be discussed, these conclusions may be modified by the severity of depression.

Carl Zimet (1979) proposed a developmental task and crisis group model of brief therapy that was quite similar to both the IDE and IPT models. Zimet described treatment of groups which extended the tenets of developmental stage theory and crisis intervention to a group format. He developed treatment groups which helped individuals deal with significant "stepping-stone" transitions throughout their life span, including midlife transition, divorce and separation, bereavement, and premarital issues. Nicholas Cummings (1991), long active in the managed care and brief therapy movement, developed a model of intermittent psychotherapy throughout the life cycle, based on a similar concept of life span development and life stage theory. Cummings likened therapeutic utilization in his approach to the approach of the family physician. The family physician deals with acute problems as they arise, and the patient returns for therapy as new problems develop. Cummings would focus treatment on the immediate disruption in life functioning, and would employ it in an individual, rather than a group format.

Cognitive models can also be quite appropriate to briefer therapy formats. Beck's *Cognitive Therapy of Depression* (Beck, Rush, Shaw, and Emery, 1979) certainly lends itself to focal therapy. Beck's therapy attempts to modify the cognitive patterns which seem associated with depression. As will be discussed below, Beck viewed cognitive patterns as causing a person to see the self, the future, and experiences in a "depressogenic" manner. Such people view themselves in a negative way, interpret ongoing experiences negatively and critically, and regard the future in a pessimistic and negative way. They display faulty information processing, arbitrarily inferring negative conclusions in the absence of evidence to support the conclusion or when the evidence is contrary to a conclusion. They overgeneralize and draw conclusions on the basis of one or more isolated incidents, relating external events to themselves when there is little basis to do so, and manifesting other such faulty cognitive patterns. Finally, Beck regards rigid views of oneself, life, other people, and the world as "schemas" which restrict full and depression-free functioning.

The theory of Alfred Adler can be applied to a cognitive perspective on psychotherapy and certainly lends itself to brief and insight-oriented approaches. The Adlerian view is that an individual may have mistaken assumptions about the world, the self, and the behavior necessary to achieve security and success, resulting in mistaken goals. This mistaken worldview consists of assumptions which have become so familiar to the patient that they seem obvious. Much like a fish in water, the person may be unaware of the assumptive world until it is brought into some contrast by the therapist's articulating and challenging it. Adler believed that mistaken views bring people into conflict with others and contribute to self-serving but socially noncontributory goals. Through processes such as the analysis of early recollections, lifestyle, and the interpretation of dreams, Adlerian therapists infer patterns of behavior. This is a process of collaboration with the patient to understand and review basic mistakes in his or her understanding of life, cause-effect relationships, and social goals.

Corsini (1981) shows how this can easily be applied to briefer therapies. A heuristic and anecdotal article discusses what he labeled "Immediate Therapy," confronting an individual on mistaken social goals in a rather intensive group setting. Corsini worked with what some might see as a very difficult patient population, prison inmates, and he found quick success, at least in some instances, using this modality. He stressed the need for collaboration and the interpersonal nature of treatment and pathology.

Marital and family therapies have as a focal point the social context within which an individual lives. Family relationships are seen as the most prominent relationships in a person's life. The systems therapists (e.g., deShazer, 1985; Haley, 1976; Cade & O'Hanlan, 1993; Croake & Olson, 1977) view symptoms as occurring in a social context. They see some difficulties requiring treatment as resulting from mistaken attempts to solve a problem. The focal point of many of the marriage and family systems approaches to therapy is the problem-maintaining nature of attempted solutions or feedback cycles, as Budman and Gurman (1988) have characterized them. As deShazer (1985) states, "the goal of therapy is not 'elimination of the symptom,' but rather, helping the client set up some conditions that allow for spontaneous achievement of the stated (or inferred) goal.... It is not that either a person has symptoms or he does not. That a certain behavior is labeled a symptom is arbitrary: In some other setting or with a different meaning attached, the same behavior would be both appropriate and normal" (p. 14). The systems therapist would attempt to focus on the context of symptom display, its social meaning, significance, and effect, and respond to it not merely in an interpersonal model, but in a systems model in which patterns of information processing and systems regulation are brought into play.

Many of the systems models come from studying the Ericksonian (e.g., Erickson and Rossi, 1981) approaches to treatment. The primary author of this text was most fortunate to spend some weeks studying with Milton Erickson in the 1970s and can attest to the power of some of these Ericksonian systems interventions. Erickson made much use of metaphor as a way to reconstrue relationships. He would often reframe behavior, recontextualizing problematic behavior and therefore effecting its occurrence. Erickson used to say in the small seminars at his home, "You want to get people to do the right things *for whatever reason.*" Although Erickson has been viewed as "really" advocating almost every theoretical orientation, it does seem that there is a tremendous focus on the social psychological aspects of human behavior in his theories. It deserves note that he served on a variety of editorial boards in anthropology as well as in medicine. Many of the family and marital schools of brief therapy that are systems focused stem from Ericksonion interventions.

Other marriage and family therapies take a more "traditional" interpersonal approach to problem solving and communication enhancement. As will be discussed, even involvement of the patient's spouse or partner in more traditional psychotherapy is likely to produce a positive benefit in treatment outcome. The brief therapy practitioner may focus on developing interpersonal skills that affect the marriage or may attempt to deal with the press of symptoms by attending carefully to the patient's marital and family context.

Other therapists focus on the time-limited nature of therapy and see the need to use a problem-solving model. Perhaps the most visible current advocate of single-session therapy is Moshe Talmon (e.g., Talmon, 1990). He conceptualizes the single session of psychotherapy as a whole and "potentially complete therapeutic intervention in and of itself." As is noted by Austad and Hoyt (1992), a guiding principle of single-session therapy is the view that the power of the therapeutic process lies within patients, and their capacity for growth should never be underestimated. Such therapy also acknowledges that small steps can make a big difference in the change process, and that more therapy is not necessarily better therapy.

The problem-solving therapist attempts to assess what is maintaining the patient's problem and what is needed to facilitate change. Though therapeutic work may not be completed during a single session, it may be initiated or redirected through other attempts to complete therapy through subsequent changes in living. Therapeutic methods include pre-session and end-of-session structuring, decreasing attachment to a patient's single view of self, and pointing out "exceptions to the rule" of the patient's symptoms, emphasizing positive behaviors and reframing or altering the context or meaning of an action or pattern. Single-session therapy has not been seen as appropriate for certain populations, including the suicidal and the psychotic.

The authors' approach to brief therapy, were it to be formally labeled, might be called therapeutic management. We believe that therapeutic outcomes should be the focus, and the therapist should coordinate the change process through whatever mechanisms appear most effective, collaborating with the patient and drawing upon feedback of success or nonsuccess to alter treatment plans. Drawing upon a host of models, including cognitive and Adlerian therapy, interpersonal therapy, biological interventions, and even single-session therapy, this approach advocates a very practical and pragmatic approach to briefly altering *patterns* of problematic behavior that impede a solution to specific problems. Therapy to alter problematic *patterns of psychosocial behavior* may include psychotherapy or may coordinate other forms of "life therapy." Such activities as the Outward Bound program for adolescents, self-help groups and parenting classes, monitoring and enhancing patients' adherence to treatment with antidepressant medicines, increasing one's level of physical activity through exercise and recreational programs, or any of a vast number of other life changes can augment and supplement the therapeutic process.

Therapeutic management can involve the use of systematic programs for addressing common problems or needs in a defined population. We advocate a pragmatic and research-based approach to symptom modification as symptoms relate to syndromes or patterns of behavior. The application of this approach to treatment, one selected for a managed care context, will, we hope, become evident in both its manifestations and its basis throughout the remainder of this book.

3

Theories of Depression

Treatment in the managed care environment requires specific knowledge about the conditions the provider is treating. Treatment planning is the core of managed care. With respect to depression, the therapist is fortunate, since there is no shortage of theories intended to illuminate and explain it. Theories range widely: from those that emphasize the biological underpinnings of depression to those that focus on its social context, from those that look at behaviors to those that explore phenomenology or emotional experience, from the old to the new, and from the more simple to the ornately complex.

Theories of depression also vary in terms of the research supporting them. Within the social and medical sciences, empirical research has always been a way to validate theoretical understanding. Some theories, by their nature, lend themselves less well than others to empirical validation or refutation. Psychoanalytic theory is one of these. Other theories may be open to empirical inquiry, but practical considerations may constrain research efforts. For example, longitudinal research is expensive, and funding is often hard to obtain for studies that will not bear fruit for years, if at all. Theories that could be investigated by life-span research, therefore, will probably not be explored empirically. Funding for studies of drug effectiveness, relevant to certain biological theories, on the other hand, might be more available from the pharmaceutical companies that produce the antidepressant medicines being investigated. In short, there is hardly a consensus on the causes of depression, and the validation for the various views is often wanting.

BIOLOGICAL THEORIES

Theories of depression can be easily divided into those that refer to biological causes and those that refer to psychological causes. Biological theories may well be historically the most accepted, and they have strong currency today. A review article by Lewis (1967) about melancholia notes that even Hippocrates proposed a biological basis for melancholia. He believed that the accumulation of "black bile and phlegm" affected one's mood state, "darkening the spirit and making it melancholic."

Many genetic studies have suggested that some mood disorders have a biological component. These studies imply that the biology of an individual, through genetic inheritance, plays a role in the etiology of depressive disorders.

Twin studies compare the rates of similar diagnoses, called the "concordance rate," for monozygotic twins, who possess identical sets of genes. There are repeated findings of a higher concordance rate in monozygotic twins than in dizygotic twins, who have a different genetic structure. In fact, a concordance rate of 63.8% for mood disorders has been observed in monozygotic twins, compared with a 14% rate for dizygotic twins (Wesner and Winokur, 1990). Adoption studies have attempted to separate genetically based susceptibility from environmental factors. Assessing the concordance rates in twins raised away from their biological parents might point toward the inheritability of certain disorders. Although all of these studies can be questioned on methodological grounds, multiple studies (e.g., Cadoret, 1978; Von Knorring, Cloninger, Bohman, and Sigvardsson, 1983) show a significant difference in concordance rates. These studies suggest that bipolar disorder very likely has, and certain forms of unipolar depression probably have, a genetic basis, and that other mood disorders may not be genetically based. Family studies acertain the ratio of ill relatives to the total number of relatives. This risk for a disorder, called the "morbid risk," appears significantly high for both bipolar and unipolar disorders.

Studies are currently under way to explore the genetic markers which may be associated with depression, such as blood group markers and DNA markers. These are very complex studies with methodological flaws, and their results have not yet been replicated.

However, they hint at a biological basis to mood disorders (see, for example, Morton, 1955; Shapiro, Block, Rafaelson, Ryder, and Svejgaard, 1976; and Hill, Wilson, Elston, and Winokur, 1988).

The theory of how biology affects depression has led to the examination of the neurotransmitters which control mood states. A comparison of depressive reactions with other diseases caused by a deficiency of such factors as vitamins or other substances prompted the theory that a deficiency of certain neurotransmitters might lead to a depressive state. This theory has been revised to hypothesize that imbalances between systems of neurotransmitters and deregulations of biochemical systems are more likely to cause depression, in view of the complexity of the brain and the subtlety of the neurochemistry of neurological functioning (e.g., Siever and Davis, 1985). In some form or in some combination, then, neurotransmitters are seen as the culprits causing depression, according to the biological theories.

There are three principal neurobiological theories of depression. The oldest has to do with norepinephrine, a catecholamine which as far back as 1929 was seen to have a function in the "fight or flight" response to threatening stimuli. In 1950 Hans Selye demonstrated the effects on norepinephrine of physiological responses to stress. An absolute or relative deficiency of this biogenic amine or of other catecholamines in certain areas of the brain was considered to cause depression (e.g., Schildkraut, 1965). Although the original formulation of the singular deficiency in catecholamine as the cause of depression has not been confirmed after closer scrutiny, there has been continuing interest in the role of norepinephrine in mood disorders.

A different biological basis was proposed in the 1970s, first by Janowsky, El-Yousef, Davis, and Sererke (1972). An imbalance between cholinergic and adrenergic activity in specific brain sites and increased cholinergic activity without a compensatory noradrenergic increase was thought to lead to depression. It had been well established that the cholinergic and adrenergic agents could affect mood states. Although the research is complex and far from clear, mood disorders do appear to involve an imbalance between these two systems, but whether this causes or merely correlates with depression is unknown.

A third and currently more fashionable hypothesis has to do with the role of serotonin. Several studies show the role of functional deficit in serotonin in depressive illness. Postmortem studies of depressed and suicidal patients found reduced levels of serotonin or its metabolites (e.g., Bourne, Bunney, and Colburn, 1968; Shure, Campes, and Eccleston, 1967; and Beskow, Gottfries, Roos, and Winblad, 1976). Decreased levels of the serotonin metabolite used in research studies have been found in the cerebral spinal fluid of depressed patients (Asberg and Bertilsson, 1979; et al.). Other studies explore the role of such biological factors as dopamine, endorphin function, and biological rhythms, including sleep and seasonal cycles.

The studies suggest that the neurotransmitters, such as norepinephrine, catecholamines, and serotonin, play a part in a depressive illness and that other biological factors may also be involved in mood disorders. Care should be taken not to draw unwarranted conclusions from these biological studies, given the complexity of the neurological systems involved. Much of this research will likely be found to have more heuristic than conclusory value. In their very thoughtful book, *Pseudoscience in Biological Psychiatry: Blaming the Body,* Colin Ross and Alvin Pam (1995) point out: "The idea of the depression as based on a biological deficit comes from the observation that depressed people are low on energy, plus bioreductionism. A severely depressed person is like a record playing at slow speed, with reduced energy, slowed movements, reduced range of body movement, slow thinking, reduced range of facial expression and little interest in things. The intuitively obvious conclusion is that the depressed person is low on something: the thinking that led to the biological deficit theories of depression is no more sophisticated than this ... the biological deficit model is based on simple reasoning, drug company marketing, and no good data. There is no scientific evidence whatsoever that clinical depression is due to any kind of biological deficit state" (p. 109).

Whether they are due to a deficiency of neurotransmitters, a correlate of other causes, or a cause itself, there are some biological differences in groups of depressed patients compared to those without mood disorders. Frontal lobe hypometabolism is seen on Positron Emission Tomography scans. Limbic changes seem to result in increased corticotropin-releasing hormone (CRH) and thyrotropin-releasing hormone (TRH). Pituitary and adrenal glands are often altered in size in depressed patients (Post, 1994). Something abnormal is going on biologically in the depressed patient, although there is more surmise than certainty as to what, why, and how.

It is clear, however, that certain forms of depression respond to antidepressant medicines. The Depression Guideline Panel, formed by the U.S. Department of Health and Human Services' Agency for Policy Care Research and composed of experts on depression, concluded that there was the clearest possible evidence that "medications have been shown to be effective in all forms of major depression," and that "patients with moderate to severe major depressive disorder are appropriately treated with medication, whether or not formal psychotherapy is also used." These conclusions are based on numerous outcome studies and a review of all current available research on treatment of depression, particularly in primary care settings. It should be recalled, however, that a *response* to biological agents does not in and of itself prove a biological *cause* for depression.

PSYCHOLOGICAL THEORIES

Often on a separate track from the biological theories, psychological theories of depression have evolved to account for the etiology, course, and psychopathology of mood disorders. Perhaps one of the earliest of these was that of Sigmund Freud. Freud's theory of psychosexual development posited distinct developmental phases: oral, anal, and phallic. Traumas or delayed development in any of these stages could cause fixations and psychopathological reactions, including depression. Abraham (1911) refined Freud's theory by focusing on the oral stage and claimed that fixations at this first developmental stage lead to depression. Rado (1928) and Melanie Klein (1934) discussed other problems and disruptions in early childhood which bring about a fixed perception of the self as helpless and powerless. Freud (1917) himself expanded his theory of the self-critical nature of depression as follows: "If one listens patiently to the many and varied self-accusations of the melancholic one cannot in the end avoid the impression that often the most violent of these are hardly at all applicable to the patient himself but that with insignificant modifications they do fit someone else, some person who the patient loves, has loved or ought to love" (p. 243).

Freud regarded the depressed patient as identifying with a lost or unavailable person, and he viewed introjected anger as an important component of depression. Aggression is the recurrent theme in the various psychoanalytic theories for most classical and neo-Freudian writers. Whether aggression is an inborn destructive drive or, in Stone's (1986) words, "a forceful, painful or destructive mode of coercing an object to the subject's will," aggression and the role of fixations are at the core of the analytic view.

Psychoanalytic theory and its most recent manifestation, object relations theory, have led to psychotherapeutic interventions for depression and other psychiatric problems. The historical influence of these views is significant. Traditional psychoanalytic therapy was fairly long-term, initially striving to uncover unconscious emotional material through free association. Refinements have focused more upon emotional catharsis, the venting and expressing of emotions, something a psychoanalytic therapist would think best done in the context of a stable, continuing, and well-boundaried relationship. The spotlight is trained upon emotional expressiveness, since emotional traumas and patterns of repressed emotional expressiveness are seen by the psychoanalyist as at the heart of depression.

While psychoanalytic therapy was developing in a more medical environment, research psychologists were developing experimental techniques for better understanding human and animal behavior. Learning theory and behavioral approaches were evolving, with operant conditioning regarded as a mechanism of behavioral control by Skinner and classical conditioning effects explored initially by Pavlov. Behavioral researchers considered an entirely different domain of data and took a very different approach from the psychoanalysts, who were more concerned with the intrapsychic level.

One approach which lent itself to treatment of depression reflected theories that viewed deficient patterns of behavioral reinforcement as affecting the depressed person. According to operant theory, behavior which is rewarded will increase in frequency and behavior which is not awarded will decrease in frequency, a process referred to as behavioral "extinction." The depressed person typically exhibits a low rate of behavioral activity, leading to the view that behavior has not been sufficiently reinforced. Peter Lewinsohn (1974) proposed a low rate of "response contingent positive reinforcement" as the cause of depression. He further suggested that deficits in the behavioral skills of the individual prevent social reinforcement. He refers to "the complex ability both to emit behaviors which are positively or negatively reinforced, and not to emit behaviors which are punished or extinguished by others." Lewinsohn developed a treatment plan which involved behavioral monitoring and deliberate behavioral change. Social skills training was added to this paradigm in later years, with assertiveness training serving as an important component in the treatment for depression.

Deficits in problem-solving skills were also seen as preventing reinforcement. Nezu (1987) noted deficits in five areas of problem solving: orienting to a problem, defining and formulating the nature of the problem, developing alternative responses, making appropriate decisions, and implementing valid possible solutions. The effect of good problem-solving skills, such as assertiveness, is to allow one to interact better with the world and to gain reinforcement or maintain reinforcers. Nezu proposed training in problem-solving skills as a component to treatment of depression.

Deficits or changes in the environment might cause a loss or lack of reinforcers, which can in turn also cause behavioral extinction and thus depression. Ferster (1966) discusses the loss of reinforceable *behavior*. A loss in a behavioral repertoire caused by sudden or profound environmental or developmental changes can lead to a loss of behaviors that might provide reinforcement. This is particularly likely if one does not have alternative behaviors that can provide reward in a new environment. In effect, all of these theories refer to a reduction in the rate or effectiveness of positive reinforcement. It should be noted that many of these theories focus on reinforcement received from others in one's *social* environment, necessitating social skills training or other interpersonal interventions in order to increase the rate of social reinforcement.

Costello (1972) discusses loss of reinforcement effectiveness. Behaviors can lose their effectiveness as a reinforcer for a variety of reasons, one of which might be satiation of reward. In layman's terms, a person can get tired of something that was previously quite enjoyable. A somewhat more complex and intriguing view is one offered by Eastman (1976), who talks about the interdependent nature of behavior, stimuli, and reinforcers. According to this theory, a loss of a reinforcer and a behavioral change can disrupt an entire reward system. Eastman explains this by analogy, "Consider a tightly stretched net, made of some elastic filament. The knots in this net represent behaviors, stimuli and reinforcers, while the filaments between them represent the interdependencies. If the single knot is excised, a large hole appears: the net effectively collapses. This represents the disruption of the relationship between the behavior, stimuli and reinforcers that Costello calls a 'loss of reinforcer effectiveness.' If the net is only loosely stretched in the first place and if there are no in-built holes (some behaviors, etc., are not interrelated with others), then the removal of one knot will only have a small effect on the total" (p. 282).

This theory has been applied to patients who have been overly invested in a limited aspect of possible rewards, for example, the mother who has found primary reward in children now grown, the retired person who has found the primary source of focus and reward in work, and others who may have "put all their eggs in one basket." The theory implies that a diversification of rewards, much akin to a diversification recommended in a financial portfolio, may provide better stability of emotional "income" in changeable times. This suggests that a multiplicity of rewarding interests can be a safeguard against depression. Loss of one interest or activity, for physical or other reasons, still allows for reinforcement from the other areas of interest.

Lewinsohn, Hoberman, Teri, and Hautzinger (1985) concluded that some of the early views might be too simplistic. Although they note that their behavioral program has been found quite effective, they think that a theory of depression should acknowledge that situational factors may be triggers, that cognitive factors may be moderators, and that clear risk factors and vulnerabilities may predispose a person toward depression in some situations. This implies that behavioral factors may be only one aspect of a depressive response.

A different behavioral model was developed by Lazarus (1968) and Wolpe (1972). They discussed how prolonged anxiety might lead to the anticipation of frustration or the expectation of nonreward. They saw continuing stress as leading to the expectation of punishment or nonreward for any behavioral output, the theory they refer to as "aversive control." Gray (1987) notes that this is very similar to the behavioral theory of condition inhibition. According to this theory, stimuli which signal that no reward is forthcoming tend to inhibit responses. An example is memories of one's deceased spouse, which serve to remind one that a person is no longer able to offer companionship and that the rewards of the marriage will never recur, regardless of one's actions.

Other forms of behavioral theory and learning theory have also been employed to understand depression. As far back as the 1920s, scientists in Pavlov's laboratory noted that training a dog to make discriminations produced reactions reminiscent of depression once the stimuli were made impossible to discriminate. For example, dogs might be conditioned quite easily to respond to the lower of two pitches of sounds, displaying no signs of unusual patterns of response. Dogs then forced to choose between two sounds so close in pitch as to defy discrimination would find the task immobilizing. The discovery that helplessness could be a learned response inspired the learned helplessness theory of depression.

In the 1960s, Seligman and Maier (1967), among others, researched the responses in animals who received inescapable shocks. Receiving an unavoidable aversive reaction in one situation led animals to fail to learn later to escape similar shocks in a situation where avoidance was possible. Seligman (1975) later developed and modified the theory of learned helplessness. He found that exposure to uncontrollable aversive events led to several responses, including motivational deficits, such as a lack of effort to learn, and cognitive deficits and deteriorations in cognitive efficiency. Emotional changes, including depression, were also observed. Later theories (Abrahmson, Seligman, and Teasdale, 1978) also noted the importance of cognitive factors in a learned helplessness model of depression. They looked at the importance of causal attributions, the degree to which one had attributed responsibility to self or others for the cause of aversive events, and the expectation of the future uncontrollability of awards.

This idea is reminiscent of the concept of locus of control, according to which people differ in the degree to which they believe that the control of rewards is exercised by external events versus more internal factors. Someone who believes that important decisions or the occurrence of rewards is controlled by such external factors as luck or fortune has a very external locus of control. The converse is the person who has the very internal locus of control, which can be summarized by a line in the poem *Invictus* (W. E. Henley) "I am the master of my fate. I am the captain of my soul." This person believes that rewards are controlled by oneself and by factors such as effort and motivation. The theory suggests that an external locus of control is more inclined to correlate with depression, given the helplessness implied by this attributional style, while an internal locus of control correlates more with freedom from depression.

Subsequent theories expanded this view to include other ways in which people might attribute causes for events in their life. Another attributional element which may be related to depression is whether one views events as resulting from stable and invariant forces or from unstable and transient factors. Whether global or specific factors were regarded as the causes of events was also investigated. These other elements of attributional style can be illustrated by various ways of viewing an event, for example, a theft: occurring due to stable factors ("Thieves will always get you"); more transient ones ("Since the mill closed down some people have turned to theft until they get real jobs"); as a result of global factors ("People are not concerned with other peoples' rights"); or very specific ones ("Thieves must target homes such as ours with no light on outside").

The evidence is mixed for the importance of attributional style in depression. Hargreaves (1985) found no differences in attributional style between depressed patients and studied controls. Brewin (1985) found an attributional style as applied to *negative* events in depressed patients. Attributional style is seen as important in other behaviors which may lead to life changes and depression. Burns and Seligman (1989) note a variety of correlates of attributional style, including health. Certain attributional patterns are likely to prompt good health maintenance behavior, and therefore good health. It appears, however, that maladaptive attributions are present with some depressed patients, but not with others (Brewin, 1989).

Rehm (1977) and Kanfer (1977) developed what might be referred to as self-control theory, a further step away from the purely behavioral. This theory focuses on three deficits in self-regulation: in self-monitoring, in self-evaluation, and in self-reinforcement. Self-monitoring deficits include a perceptual style in which there is a focus on negative events that follow behavior, to the exclusion of positive events. This perceptual style filters out positive perceptions and amplifies awareness of negative events. The second deficit in self-monitoring is the focus on immediate rather than longer-term rewards for behavior. A person exercising, for example, might notice the immediate reward of fatigue or muscle discomfort rather than the longer-term consequences of good health and fitness.

A self-evaluation occurs when there is a comparison between observed performance and a standard for performance. A self-evaluation of a deficiency refers to a gap between observed and desired levels of functioning. Deficits in self-evaluation can occur in two ways. The first is in the observation of performance. One might have made an unrealistic appraisal of the proportion of errors committed, for example, or underestimate one's productivity, in effect judging oneself too critically. The other deficiency is in comparing one's behavior to an unrealistic internalized standard. When the depressed person indicates that "I am not what I should be" he or she may be unrealistic or mistaken regarding how he or she is or should be. An example of this is perfectionism, in which a person believes that his or her work is flawed and that his or her performance is inadequate, when by any objective standard the performance was *more* than adequate.

Finally, self-control theory discusses deficiencies in self-reinforcement. Goals which are unattainable make reinforcement unlikely. Perfectionistic excessive goals for reward attainment are an example. A person with perfection as a goal may provide self-reward only for perfect performance rather than "merely" for performance which was more than satisfactory. Delaying a reinforcement until an outcome is completely achieved rather than providing incremental reinforcement as one progresses toward a larger goal is another deficiency in self-reinforcement.

Studies on achievement orientation in children show that patterns of self-reinforcement are correlated with achievement orientation (e.g., McClelland, 1961). Children given a task, for example bowling, are given the opportunity to reinforce themselves with dimes or M&M candies if they have performed up to standards they see as appropriate for each frame bowled. Responses will generally cluster into groups of those who set high standards for self-reward, those who establish more moderate ones, and those who have a very low threshold for reinforcement. Some children will take a dime or a candy each time they bowl, regardless of their success. Others will delay a reward until they have bowled a strike or a spare, requiring excellent performance before any award occurs. Others will set some standard, for example knocking over six or seven pins, and then reward themselves. Some studies suggest that it is the middle group that reflects the highest degrees of achievement orientation and achievement in school.

COGNITIVE THEORIES

Cognitive theories of depression and psychopathology are much in vogue today and a focus of current research and writing. These theories have their origins in the work of Adler and Kelly and have received attention more recently from Albert Ellis, David Meichenbaum, and Aaron Beck. The theories generally suggest that it is the thoughts intervening between a stimulus and an emotional reaction that moderate and determine the reaction. While most people believe that a stimulus leads automatically to a reaction, Albert Ellis (1962) points out that an activating event (A) does not cause a reaction, or consequence (C), without an intervening belief (B). Ellis' rational emotive therapy focused predominately on changing the beliefs in order to change the consequences of the emotional reaction. Ellis' books, such as *A New Guide to Rational Living* (Ellis and Harper, 1975), were very popular among the lay public and were found helpful by many professionals. Rational emotive therapy is still actively practiced, although Ellis himself has modified his theory and now calls it rational emotive behavior theory. He has long made use of behavioral techniques, particularly self-reinforcement, in the therapeutic process (Ellis, 1993).

According to Aaron Beck (1967, 1976), a psychiatrist who studied with Ellis, there are idiosyncratic patterns of thought in depressed patients which not only correlate with, but might be seen as causing, depression. Cognitive behavior therapy is a school of treatment, developed by Beck but with a long philosophical history, which evolved from this theory. This therapy attempts to modify the thinking behaviors, or cognitions, of depressed patients.

According to cognitive behavior therapy, there are three aspects of disturbed thinking: negative automatic thoughts, systematic logical errors in thinking, and "depressogenic schemas." Negative automatic thoughts are those which occur so quickly that they may not even be perceived by the individual and which contribute to depression in depressed patients. Those with depression usually believe that they, personally, are inadequate to deal with the challenges they face. They view the external world as impossibly hard, demanding, exacting, and unforgiving. They believe that the future holds no hope. These "automatic thoughts," or assumptions about the world, are seen as one aspect of the cognitive cause of depression.

Beck discusses several types of systematic logical errors in thinking. *Arbitrary inference* takes place when an individual makes conclusions from insufficient data. There is no evidence, or insufficient evidence, to support these conclusions, or there may even be evidence to contradict them. An extreme example of this is found in severe depression, including psychotic depression where patients may even believe that they are responsible for wars or natural disasters. *Selective abstraction* refers to focusing on one detail out of many, ignoring aspects of the context of the situation and understanding the whole situation or experience on the basis of this one detail. *Overgeneralization* refers to a pattern of drawing a general rule or conclusion merely because one incident, or rare incidents, have occurred. Attempting to apply these conclusions about unique events to all or perhaps unrelated situations can result from this. *Magnification* and *minimization* refer to errors in evaluating the magnitude or significance of an occurrence. *Personalization* refers to the tendency to assume that external events are related to the person even when there is no evidence for this. *Absoluteness*, or *dichotomous thinking*, is the tendency to think in black and white categories, an "all-or-none" cognitive approach.

Depressogenic schemas are the third category of idiosyncratic cognitive styles in depressed patients. Beck (1964) defines these as "a structure for screening, coding and evaluating impinging stimuli." These schemas can be seen as dimensions that the person considers relevant or meaningful. Beck says that "the schema constitutes the basis for screening out, differentiating and coding the stimuli that confront the individual. He categorizes and evaluates his experiences through a matrix of schema" (p. 13). Examples of such schemas include dependency, social isolation, and incompetence.

Young (1989) has developed a questionnaire to assess these schemas, finding this particularly relevant to patients with personality disorders. His work indicates 15 major schematic categories, separate dimensions upon which a person is overly attentive for signals. Signals along these dimensions may cause patients to conclude that they are vulnerable or insufficient in the way defined by the schema. An example is a schema of abandonment and loss, where a person looks for signals of rejection and feels inadequate or vulnerable if any such signal occurs. It should be noted that the schemas imply a form of hypervigilance. A person with a borderline personality disorder, for example, might be overly attentive to signals of rejection or abandonment, reacting at a much lower threshold for response than might be the case for other people. Such a patient might infer rejection from the most subtle of cues, unfortunately often creating rejection by excessive reactions.

A cognitive-behavioral approach explores the cognitive contribution to depression in an almost mechanical way. Other "cognitive theories" seem more to emphasize the *phenomenology* of individuals, their subjective reality, and the *meaning* of their experiences to them. The authors consider the theory of Alfred Adler (1956, 1964, 1978) to be such a cognitive and social-psychologically based theory with much relevance to the treatment of a variety of disorders, including depression. Adler believed that individuals strive to attain a subjectively conceived goal of success within a social context. This subjective goal has meaning within a person's view of the social world. This "assumptive world" is a fairly consistent phenomenological reality for the individual and produces consistent patterns of action or personality, called a "lifestyle." To the degree to which the person's view of the world and his or her personal goals are consonant with social functioning and support social contribution, the person will be socially both "reinforced" and "reinforcing." Adlerian theory, therefore, sees depression, which appears to be an intrapsychic problem, as also interpersonal in nature.

Within this view, pathological responses may be reinforced by the person's "worldview," or appropriate reactions may be limited by the person's mistaken "lifestyle." An example of this is the view of the world as a dangerous place, filled with challenges a person is unable to overcome independently, where the only hope for survival lies in convincing powerful others of one's "goodness" in order to evoke vital caretaking from those who hold the keys to safety. A person with this view might have a goal of "succeeding" by being more "good" than others, a goal of righteousness which may be excessive, inflexible, and even in conflict with more effective and appropriate interpersonal behavior. A lack of assertiveness and even martyr-like suffering may seem to be appropriate ways to pursue one's mistaken goal. This behavior might simultaneously reinforce the self-fulfilling prophecy of the world withholding satisfaction, since it is likely not to be reinforcing and may even be aversive to others. Treatment endeavors to challenge this worldview and to encourage the development of more group-relevant than self-relevant goals. This can result in a greater degree of group identification, social involvement, and social–and thus psychological– reward.

PSYCHOSOCIAL AND INTERPERSONAL THEORIES

While some theories focus on the biological aspects of depression and others on the psychological components to mood disorders, yet another dimension of theory and research explores psychosocial and interpersonal explanations for depression. Some of these psychosocial theories are based on correlational studies which show that various life events, circumstances, and differences tend to correlate with depression.

The research on life events, particularly negative events and associations between loss and depression, seems significant for an understanding of depression. The research suggests that social and interpersonal factors, rather than merely biological factors or individual behavioral or cognitive factors, play a role in the onset and persistence of depression. Dohrenwend, Shrout, Link, Martin, and Skodol (1986) found that depressed patients, when compared with community controls, had significantly more negative events in the year prior to onset of depression. These events were in three areas: fateful loss events, such as a house fire or a loss of income; physical illness or injury; and events disruptive to the patient's social support network, especially the death of a spouse.

Other researchers, such as Lewinsohn, Hoberman, and Rosen-baum (1988), and Brown, Bifulco, and Harris (1987), show associations between stressors and depression. These studies lead to the conclusion that most people who experience major negative life events do not become depressed, but that those who become depressed have often had such negative events. This suggests some comparative contribution of biological and psychological factors, on the one hand, and external and largely social occurrences, on the other.

Gender differences in depression raise similar questions about causation. More women than men get depressed, statistically by as much as a two-to-one ratio. There is some suggestion that a biological basis for depression is more common in women than in men, but the evidence seems very weak and contradictory when the research is closely reviewed. Aneshensel, Frerichs, and Clark (1981) for example, note that the rates of depression are greater only for married and employed women, suggesting that social and cultural factors, more than just gender, may be involved. Radloff (1975) saw the socialization of women as limiting the ranges of socially sanctioned responses available to them. He suggested that learned helplessness resulting from such socialization might lead to depression. Many feminist authors (e.g., Brown and Liss-Levinson, 1981) are quick to point out the cultural differences between genders which may negatively affect women. Depression can certainly be seen as resulting from such factors as reduced income, increased risk for violence, and other causes of limited rewards and reinforcers.

There are also different prevalence rates for depression for different ages. The incidence rate for depression appears to rise shortly before puberty, to remain high between ages 25 and 44, and then to decline slightly (Weissman & Myers, 1978). The initial incident of depression occurs at a younger age in women, and the greatest incidence is for women under age 35. The risk for depression then decreases. The peak rates for men occur somewhat later, in the 45-to-65-year range. Those with a bipolar mood disorder seem to have an average age of onset in the late 20s. Unipolar depression has a peak average age of onset in the middle to late 30s. The different rates of medical utilization, different symptom displays in children, and different diagnostic criteria addressed in the research studies mean that such prevalence data should be regarded as somewhat tentative.

There is also evidence that socioeconomic status affects rates of depression. There are very consistent reports that depression is more often found in those of lower, rather than higher, socioeconomic groups (Brown and Harris, 1978). An exception is found in bipolar disorder, which is more prevalant in people of higher socioeconomic status. Studies show that married women with young children, with lower income and lower status jobs, are more likely to become significantly depressed than those in other circumstances. Married working-class women with more than two children of any age also appear to be a group at significant risk for depression.

The correlation between socioeconomic status and depression does not necessarily indicate causation. It is plausible that those who are depressed behave in ways less likely to gain social reward, and that therefore they are more likely to be constrained from economic advancement. Other social theories suggest that social reinforcement is less available to some groups who are economically deprived, and that this causes depression. Regardless of the causes or implications, sociological data do tend to correlate socioeconomic status and gender with depression and other health problems. Women and those of lower socioeconomic status are significantly more likely to be depressed.

Depressed people are shown in many research studies to have smaller and less supportive social networks than nondepressed people. Studies show that there are fewer other people involved in depressed people's lives (e.g., Pattison, de Francisco, Wood, Frazier, and Crowder, 1975). Some studies show fewer nonfamily contacts for depressed as compared with nondepressed populations (Brugha et al., 1982). Other studies (e.g., Gotlib and Lee, 1989) show that people with depression engage in fewer family activities than do controls. This research seems to indicate that there is less social support because the depressed person is less socially active, but it has also been argued that depression *precedes* social inactivity. Some might view this correlational data as signifying that depression causes one to interact less with other people, not that it arises from diminishing social involvement and support. There does seem to be a connection, even if the direction of causation is still unclear.

Another body of research indicates that the relationships of the depressed person are less supportive, not merely less social, than the relationships of the nondepressed, or at least that they are perceived to be less supportive. This implies that the world of the depressed person is less socially supportive than for the more buoyant (e.g., Billings, Cronkite, and Moos, 1983). Some studies show that low levels of social support precede depression (Cutrona, 1984; Monroe, Imhoff, Wise, and Harris, 1983). The lack of social support, as assessed on intake, has even been found to correlate with remission (Billings and Moos, 1985). Billings and Moos have also argued that depression tends to affect intimate relationships more than superficial ones. In other words, the depressed person might maintain some effectiveness in less close social relationships, such as at work or with casual acquaintances, but suffer more distress and dysfunction in intimate and involved relationships, as with the spouse or family.

A low level of social support is also likely to be amplified by the negative interaction patterns of the depressed patient. Some studies suggest that the depressed patient is not merely responding to a situation of impoverished social support or fewer supportive people in his or her life, but behaving in ways that cause people to be both less present and less supportive. Gotlib and Asarnow (1979) found depressed patients to be less skillful at solving interpersonal problems. Gotlib and Robinson (1982) have also found that the depressed person speaks slowly and monotonously, maintains less eye contact, and uses awkward hand movements. Blumberg and Hokanson (1983) found the content of conversations of depressed people to be far more self-focused and negatively toned than that of nondepressed people.

The clear implication is that depression is exacerbated or maintained by the behavior of the depressed person, which alienates other people and prevents social reward. Studies show that both the content and the form of communication by the depressed person tend to cause distress, discomfort, and irritability in the receiver of the communication (Coyne, 1976). The depressed person apparently interacts in ways which are aversive to others. Hammen and Peters (1978), using transcripts of conversations with depressed patients, found a negative emotional reaction on the part of subjects reading them which was not present as they read transcripts of conversations with nondepressed people. Boswell and Murray (1981) observed the same reactions from research subjects to audiotapes of depressed patients.

This leaves unresolved the question of whether a deficit of social skills is an artifact of depression or the cause of depression. This has treatment implications, since social skills training might be less effective in treating depression if the deficit in social skills was only a transitory reaction to depression which was in fact caused by unrelated or far more important factors. If so, social skills which are assessed as deficient in depressed people might tend spontaneously to return to a more functional level in response to antidepressant medicines or other treatments not emphasizing social-skills building. Lewinsohn (1986), however, has found that social skills training is effective in treatment of depression, and such intervention implies that social behavior, in fact, maintains, exacerbates, or causes at least some depressive problems.

Marital status and discord have been another subject area for research. Depression seems to correlate with marital discord. In fact, one study showed that in 30% of couples experiencing marital discord, one spouse was clinically depressed (Waring, Patton, and Wister, 1990). Some studies show that marital distress can lead to depression. Paykel and colleagues (1969) found that arguments and increased conflicts with the spouse preceded a depressive event. Brown and Harris (1978) concluded that a lack of a confiding and intimate relationship with a husband or partner was one of the primary factors associated with depression in women.

Other studies suggest that depression can lead to marital discord. Depression affects others, particularly spouses (Claussen and Yarrow, 1955; Marks and Hammen, 1982). Depressed patients and their spouses perceive their marriages as tense and angry (Gotlib and

Whiffen, 1991). Studies of spouses of bipolar patients, usually very severely disordered in their behavior, show that more than half of the spouses without a mood disorder wish they hadn't married at all (Targum, Dibble, Davenport, and Gershon, 1981). There is much evidence that interactions with depressed persons are aversive to other people.

There is also a theory that marital problems can affect the course of treatment. Sims (1977) found that patients whose depressive symptoms seemed to have been precipitated by marital discord had the poorest treatment outcomes. Hinchliffe, Hooper, and Roberts (1978) and Rush, Shaw, and Khatami (1980) showed that increased rates of success in treatment were achieved by involving a spouse in conjoined treatment for the depressed patient. An interesting study by Vaughn and Leff (1976) measured the degree of emotion expressed by a spouse. Those who expressed their often critical emotions clearly and frequently were more likely to produce relapse in partners than were the spouses of those who were low in expressed emotion. Marital treatment has been found to be effective in the outpatient treatment of major depression, either with or without the use of antidepressants (Hafner, 1994).

Early interpersonal experiences have been found to predispose one to depression. Brown (1961) noted that the death of a parent seems to be one such factor. This is contradicted by some other studies, however. Bifulco, Brown, and Harris (1987) note that the studies that correct for the quality of the post-loss parental care seem to explain some of the contradictory results. According to their conclusions, parental care following the loss of a parent may be somewhat deficient. They maintain that the vulnerability to depression from those who lose a parent during youth arises from the lack of good parental care rather than merely from the experience of parental loss. Breier et al. (1988) showed that the death of a parent, combined with poor parenting following this and with having a first-degree relative with emotional problems, accounted for much of the variance in assigning individuals to groups experiencing adult pathology as compared to normals.

Raskin, Boothe, Reatig, Schulterbrandt, and Odle (1971) found depressed patients rate their parents as less positively involved in their activities as children, less loving, less affectionate, and more negatively controlling. Jacobson, Fasman, and DiMascio (1975) found that depressed patients reported more parental rejection, greater discord, and less parental affection, again indicating a connection between psychosocial developmental events and adult depression. It should be noted that these ratings were completed by patients both after the onset of depression and as adults. Some have suggested that there is a filtering of positive memories during the course of depression (e.g., Bower, 1981) and that depressed patients may be inclined to take a dim view not only of their current circumstances, but also of the future and the past. Mosak (1971) observed that early recollections change after effective therapy. It is important also to recall that these studies refer to a patient's perceptions of parental deficiencies and do not establish the fact of deficient parenting. These ratings do not allow one validly to conclude that parental behavior directly causes depression, even if some theorists encourage that conclusion.

SYSTEMS MODELS

General systems theory explores the reciprocal influences of component parts as they interact within a system. The theory posits that all systems have interacting component parts, and that there are rules or principles which govern system functioning. According to this theory (von Bertalanffy, 1968) all systems, from a toaster to the Department of Defense, have common characteristics. Self-regulating feedback mechanisms are among those structures common to all systems. According to this view, if activities exceed a given standard, then corrective measures within the system return it to the previous level of functioning. This causes a stable state, or homeostasis, in system functioning.

Although some developments in systems thought have modified this view somewhat, its initial metaphor of a thermostat seems appropriate to illustrate self-regulatory feedback. According to a thermostatic model of systems regulation, sensors assess whether or not an optimal temperature is present and, based on sensory feedback, exert control over system components. If the room is too cold, the thermostat causes energy to be added to heating elements until a preset temperature has been achieved, and then to cease providing energy. In this model, components interact to affect each other. More "traditional" nonsystems views of cause and effect do not apply. Here, an entity may be simultaneously both an effect and a cause, much as if a thermostat controls a distant furnace, while the furnace controls the actions of the thermostat.

In primary medicine, all systems of the body are reviewed when assessing a patient. One ailing system affects the entire body, and all the systems of the body affect any given system. The most effective medicine is practiced by those who not only have a specialized focus of medical care, but can also attend to the interaction of body systems.

General systems theory is also applied to social systems, including the most elementary ones, such as a family or a couple, and more complex ones, such as a society or a large organization. General systems theory has been applied to psychopathology, where the emphasis has been on treating the system. The entity of the family or some other social context becomes the "patient." The focus is not merely on the symptomatic person who exists within the system.

According to this theory, individuals and families may both vary in their ability to deal with the diverse demands and stresses of daily life. The ability to thrive is determined by a host of factors, including the environment within which the system exists and the resources available to it, whether that "system" be a person or a family. If the entity having difficulties in coping is the family, such family dysfunction can lead to the maintenance or reinforcement of depression in an individual by the system. According to this wider perspective, it would be acknowledged that a depressed individual has an effect upon other family members, who may, often out of the best of motivations, reinforce or exacerbate the depression. An example of this is the student who is discouraged about performance in college. Parents responding to this by "support" which minimizes the importance of academic achievements or even of college itself, may tend subtly to communicate the expectation that the student will not succeed in college, inadvertently reinforcing low expectations for success on his or her part.

Other views hold family systems to be causative of problems, rather than merely maintaining or exacerbating them (e.g., Bowen, 1981). An example of this is the child who develops a somatoform disorder and spends less time at school and more at home, this seeming to occur after the mother's onset of depression. Here, the mother's depression may cause stress for the child, or it may alleviate her symptoms to have the child remain in her care, providing some interpersonal contact and thus support. The special attention on the part of the mother may also reinforce the child's symptoms.

Many family therapists view the identified patient as expressing dysfunction in the family. The depressed patient thus might be seen as expressing the mood disorder for the entire family, just as a generous member of a normal family may express the family's generosity. The focus of intervention is the family system dysfunction, not the symptom of system dysfunction seen in the depressed individual.

SUMMARY

In summary, there is much disagreement and there are many opinions about the causes of depression. Some theories advocate the importance of biological factors, which are seen as producing secondary psychological symptoms. Other theories explore the variability of depressive responses among individuals and conclude that biological factors alone are insufficient to account for depression. Such more psychological theories regard biological factors as necessary, but not sufficient, to cause depression and consider psychological factors—be they behavioral, cognitive, or interpersonal—as necessary, concomitant, or even exclusive causes. Other theories explore the sociocultural foundation of psychopathology, including depression, and attend to the context within which the depressed person lives. These theories point to the predominantly interpersonal context as affecting the course and perhaps the occurrence of symptoms of pathology, such as depression. While the theories described here are only a sample of the many theories relevant to depression, they illustrate the range of approaches and research.

4

Diagnosis of Depression and Depressive States

Not only is there much disagreement regarding the sources of depression, but it seems quite clear that the term "depression" can refer to many different states, conditions, and specific diagnoses. Depression varies from the mild to severe, from the psychotic to the nonpsychotic, and various depressive conditions differ both qualitatively and quantitatively. Further, research has suggested different treatment approaches for differing depressive diagnoses, with certain diagnoses calling for one therapeutic response and others failing to respond to such interventions. Managed care requires treatment planning that depends upon diagnosis and outcome assessment, which is the measurement of changes in a diagnosed condition. Accurate diagnosis of depression is therefore of vital importance.

DEFINITIONS OF DEPRESSION

It is increasingly clear, however, what depression is not. Depression is not simple sadness or bereavement. Depression goes far beyond merely a sad or depressed mood, and it differs from sadness or unhappiness in a variety of ways. In April 1993, the Agency for Health Care Policy and Research (AHCPR), an agency of the U. S. Department of Health and Human Services, published the Clinical Practice Guidelines for Depression, based on the views of a team of experts on depressive disorders. Though designed primarily for guidance in primary medical care, the Guidelines offer an excellent review of the consensus of thought on disorders of mood. According to the panel, there is clear evidence for the following statement:

> Depressive disorders should not be confused with the depressed or sad mood that normally accompanies specific life experiences—particularly losses or disappointments. Mood disorders involve disturbances in emotional, cognitive, behavioral and somatic regulation. The clinical depression or a mood disorder is a syndrome (a constellation of signs and symptoms) that is not a normal reaction to life's difficulties. A sad or depressed mood is only one of many signs and symptoms of a clinical depression. In fact, the mood disturbance may include apathy, anxiety, or irritability in addition to or instead of sadness; also, the patient's interest or capacity for pleasure and enjoyment may be markedly reduced. Not all clinically depressed patients are sad, and many sad patients are not clinically depressed. (p. 17)

DIAGNOSTIC CRITERIA

DSM-IV

The citation above means that depression is different from normal bereavement, disappointment, or grief, although these conditions may be a focus of treatment. The current diagnostic nomenclature is found in the fourth edition of the *Diagnostic and Statistical Manual of Mental Disorders,* or *DSM-IV,* published by the American Psychiatric Association (1994) and endorsed by most mental health professional groups in North America. The manual also indicates that depression must be an emotional reaction. Depression cannot be diagnosed if symptoms are due to a medical or physical condition or are a result of a reaction to substances.

Substance reactions can occur from a variety of sources. A person may be intoxicated by certain substances and display symptoms of depression or mania, or may have disturbances in mood during withdrawal from substances. Alcohol, amphetamines or related substances, hallucinogens, inhalants, cocaine, sedatives, and other such substances can produce disturbances of mood during the intoxication stage. Withdrawal from these may also cause disorders of mood.

As with nonprescribed substances, some medicines and environmental toxins can invoke mood symptoms, and there are a wide range of medicines prone to this effect. Accurate diagnosis demands that these factors be considered. Psychotropic medicines, such as antidepressants or benzodiazepams, can cause a host of idiopathic reactions and effect mood in unexpected ways. Medicines such as antiparkinsonian medications, antihypertensives and anticonvulsants, cardiac medications, and even oral contraceptives, muscle relaxants, and steroids can cause disruptions of mood in some people. Even exposure to some volatile substances, such as gasoline or paint, organophosphate insecticides, or carbon monoxide may cause mood symptoms. Such a mood disorder would not qualify as an emotionally caused depressive problem. The diagnosis would be that of a substance-induced disorder of mood, not depression *per se.* The depression is a factor of the diagnosis but secondary to the specific prescription or toxin.

DSM-IV also proscribes the diagnosis of depression or bipolar disorder when either is known to arise from a medical condition. These have diagnoses separate from those for depression or other disorders of mood. Between 25 and 40% of individuals with certain neurological conditions develop a marked depressive disturbance at some point during the course of the illness (*DSM-IV,* p. 368). Particularly with such conditions as Parkinson's disease, Huntington's disease, multiple sclerosis, Alzheimer's disease, and stroke there is a high risk for a medically induced disorder of mood. Metabolic conditions, such as vitamin B^{12} deficiency, endocrine conditions, such as thyroid or parathyroid disease, and autoimmune conditions, such as lupus erythematosus, and even certain viral infections, such as mononucleosis, can affect mood. Cancers, particularly cancer of the pancreas, can cause a disorder of mood, as can cerebral vascular disease. If a medical condition is seen as the cause of depression, a diagnosis is given which reflects that the mood disorder is secondary to a medical condition, not an emotionally based condition.

There are various diagnostic conceptualizations of depression. The predominant one, and the one clearly guiding health care today, is contained in *DSM-IV,* where a diagnostic system divides those disorders of mood which are not due to substances or other medical conditions into qualitative and quantitative categories. Qualitative categories include major depressive and bipolar disorder, which are viewed as different conditions. Although there is much disagreement as to whether the differences are quantitative or qualitative, there are clear differences in the degree if not the nature of symptoms between dysthymic disorder and major depressive disorder. Bipolar I and bipolar II disorders are more severe and debilitating than cyclothymic disorder, which is a less severe display of a bipolar disease.

Major Mood Disorders

Formal diagnosis involves reference to the *DSM-IV,* which contains specific criteria for diagnoses and their elements. The building blocks, or elements, of diagnoses in the *DSM-IV* are the *episodes.* These are the major depressive episode, manic episode, mixed episodes, and hypomanic episodes. Episodes are to be distinguished from the baseline level of functioning for an individual. For example, a *major depressive episode* usually develops over days to weeks. There may be a period before such episodes with milder depressive or anxiety symptoms. The essential feature of a major depressive episode is a period of at least two weeks in which there is either depressed mood or the loss of interest or pleasure in nearly all activities. In children and adolescents, irritability may be substituted for sadness as a predominant mood. Additional symptoms must be drawn from a list that includes physical changes such as with appetite, activity level, psychomotor activity, and energy reductions, as well as emotional reactions of worthlessness and guilt, thoughts of death or suicide, and impairments in thinking, concentrating, or making decisions.

A *manic episode* is defined by a distinct period of at least one week in which there is an abnormally persistent, expansive, elevated, or irritable mood. A manic episode includes a number of symptoms somewhat opposite to those of a depressive episode. A manic episode is to be distinguished from a *hypomanic episode*, which has identical, but less severe characteristic symptoms. A manic episode is sufficiently severe to cause marked impairment in social and occupational functioning, perhaps to the point of requiring hospitalization. A hypomanic episode is not sufficiently severe as to cause this level of dysfunction.

A final "building block" to diagnosis of depression is the *mixed episode,* in which there is a period of at least a week in which some criteria of both manic and depressive episodes are present each day. The mixed episode usually involves rapidly alternating moods, with agitation and dysfunction of a magnitude sufficient to disrupt occupational or social functioning or to necessitate hospitalization. These episodes often also include psychotic symptoms.

There are two forms of bipolar disorder, conveniently labeled bipolar I and bipolar II. Bipolar I is distinguished from bipolar II by the presence of one or more manic or mixed episodes. With a bipolar II disorder there is at least one hypomanic episode currently or historically, but there can never have been a manic episode or a mixed episode.

Major depressive disorder merely refers to having a major depressive episode. The diagnosis of major depressive disorder, single episode, is given when there is one such episode. If there are two or more major episodes, a diagnosis of major depressive disorder, recurrent, is given.

Dysthymia and Cyclothymia

There are less severe forms of both depressive and bipolar disorders. The less severe dimension of depressive disorder is called *dysthymic disorder,* a chronic depressed mood which has lasted at least two years (one year in children) with at least two of six specified symptoms, such as an appetite or sleep problem.

The *cyclothymic disorder* is similar to a bipolar disorder in the frequent and marked shifts in mood, but these mood shifts do not meet the criteria of major depressive, manic, or mixed episodes during at least the first two years. This disorder also has a chronic course following an insidious onset.

Other Mood Disorders

These diagnoses are not necessarily mutually exclusive. In fact, the presence of dysthymic disorder places one more at risk for a major depressive disorder, even though they are diagnostically separate. An increased risk for a bipolar disorder has also been noted in those who have already received a diagnosis of cyclothymic disorder.

There are subgroups to these diagnoses, noted by "*specifiers*." In *DSM-IV*, these specifiers are "provided to increase diagnostic specificity and create more homogeneous subgroups, assist in treatment selection, and improve prediction of prognosis." (*DSM-IV*, p. 375). Specifiers include indications of severity, whether or not there were psychotic features, and whether or not conditions are in remission. One such specifier is *catatonic features*, where the clinical picture is characterized by marked psychomotor disturbance which may reach a point of immobility or excessive motor activity referred to as catatonia.

The *melancholic features* specifier refers to a loss of interest and/or pleasure in all or almost all activities or an inability to react to stimuli which are usually pleasurable. These melancholic features are usually more pronounced in the morning and correlate with certain patterns of sleep. *Atypical features* include the capacity for moods to brighten in response to positive events, as well as weight gain and increased sleep. The specifier of a *postpartum onset* refers to major depressive episodes which occur within four weeks after delivery of a child and can involve any of the disorders of mood. *Seasonal patterns* refer to occurrence of any of the episodes noted above in relationship to certain times of the year, usually winter, with full remission occurring at other times of the year, usually spring. Finally, the specifiers *with rapid cycling* refers to the rapidity with which moods cycle in a bipolar state.

DSM-IV also notes some depressive reactions that do not meet the criteria for a major depressive disorder. The diagnosis of a depressive disorder, not otherwise specified (NOS), and a bipolar disorder NOS is given in cases where most, but not all, of the diagnostic criteria for these conditions have been met.

An *adjustment reaction* is a response to a specific event that is in excess of what might be anticipated. Symptoms must develop within three years of the onset of the stressor and cause marked distress in excess of what would be expected or cause significant impairment in social or occupational functioning. An adjustment disorder with depressed mood can be diagnosed for such episodes of depression which abate within six months once the stressor or its consequences have stopped. Finally, certain life situations produce depressive reactions that may require clinical attention, even though an individual has no mental disorder related to the problem. Relational problems or bereavement would be examples of this.

Other Considerations in Diagnosis of Depression

While diagnosis is certainly important for specificity and, as discussed below, is a vital component of managed care, there are disagreements regarding the diagnosis of depression. Costello (e.g., 1993) has certainly been one of the more thoughtful researchers and theorists in the area of depression. He notes, "There is considerable confusion among researchers and clinicians about the nature of experiential and behavioral disorders and this seems to be because thinking in terms of syndromes is to bite off more than they can chew." Costello has proposed that attention initially be placed more on symptoms of depression rather than on more elaborate syndromes, as is done in the current *DSM.*

Kendell (1988) expresses some similar concerns:

> We have learnt how to make reliable diagnoses but we still have no adequate criteria for their validity, and this achievement focuses attention on the failures. We draw the boundaries between one syndrome and another, between illness and normality, in widely different places using widely different criteria and we have no adequate means of deciding which is right, or even which is preferable for any given project.

Brown (1991) in a thoughtful paper looks at the importance of threshold levels for establishing a "case" of depression. Reconsidering studies in which a "case" of depression was diagnosed for those displaying four specific symptoms, and comparing these to "borderline cases" in which fewer symptoms are present, casts a very different light on the research. These levels of threshold for diagnosis become important particularly when one is exploring etiology and response to types of treatment.

Clark and Watson (1991) and others show the overlap between depression and anxiety, suggesting an underlying disposition not to experience merely depression, but a variety of negative emotions, or negative affect (NA). This concept is similar to Eysenck and Eysenck's (1968) view of "neuroticism." Kleinman and Good (1985) show that dysphoria, sadness, hopelessness, and unhappiness have dramatically different forms and meanings in different societies. The prevalence rate of depression using the *DSM-IV* criteria varies greatly across cultures, but there is a cross-cultural similarity in bodily symptoms of what appears to be depression. Somatization, the expression of personal or interpersonal distress in the idiom of bodily complaints, appears more reflective of depression in some cultures than in others. Jenkins, Kleinman, and Good (1991) state that "the models of depression based on studies of inpatients and outpatients in western psychiatric settings tend to emphasize a picture of depression that is not the main one in nonwestern societies (where the vast majority of the world's population and the most depressed live)" (p. 7).

Other authors discuss the difference between melancholic and nonmelancholic depressions, drawing a distinction between those patients with or without the primary presentation of physical manifestations, or "vegetative symptoms," of depression as compared to those with the more behavioral or mood-based depressions. It could well be that *DSM-IV* provides more the illusion of agreement and understanding than actual consensus and understanding, but at least it does provide a common referent for "depression" and other mood disorders.

TESTS FOR DEPRESSION

There are no medical tests which can diagnose depression in an individual, even though a few studies show different group averages for depressed as compared to nondepressed patients on a variety of measures. Diagnosis is made through psychiatric or psychological evaluation, primarily through interviewing and testing. It is generally agreed that unstructured interviews are less reliable than structured approaches for identifying syndromes and making diagnoses, although Costello (1993) suggests that this view is more mythical than real.

Structured interviews usually entail the use of instruments or protocols for general diagnostic evaluation. Depression may be a finding of a multiaxial diagnosis, such as the Present State Examination (PSE) (Wing, Birley, Cooper, Graham, and Isaacs, 1967) attempts to provide. The ninth edition of this form defines 140 symptoms, ranging from incoherence to tension. These symptoms are specifically defined in the manual, and interviewer training and familiarity are important for accurate use of the format. The interviewer determines if the symptoms have been present in the last month, and these ratings are cross-validated by additional analysis, using tapes or transcripts. This process helps confirm that "cases" of depression, or other diagnoses, exist. The Schedule for Affective Disorders and Schizophrenia (SADS) (Endicott and Spitzer, 1978) provides a similar structured format, although it varies in its degree of symptom definition.

Although behavioral rating scales and ancillary informants are sometimes used, testing is the predominant technique used to supplement or validate an interview. Self-report inventories, questionnaires completed by the patient, are used more often than the projective techniques for a host of psychometric, economic, and perhaps "political" reasons. The most often employed general clinical diagnostic tests are the Minnesota Multiphasic Personality Inventory (MMPI) (Hathaway and McKinley, 1942) and the Millon Clinical Multiaxial Inventory (MCMI) (Millon, 1983). These tests assess broad dimensions of personal functioning. Both provide the opportunity for narrative computer interpretation as well as statistical scoring through the test publishers. The narrative reports include the test authors' assessment of the likely significance of elevated scores at certain threshold points. Diagnostic conclusions or alternatives are often mentioned. The authors of these tests and professional associations such as the American Psychological Association advise that the tests alone cannot provide a reliable diagnosis. Additional diagnostic evaluation is essential for accuracy and validity of diagnosis.

It should be remembered that although psychological testing has many strengths, it also has many limitations. It provides hypotheses which need to be confirmed against other sources of diagnostic data, such as interview impressions, knowledge of medical status, information about patient history, and behavioral reports. Further, testing is somewhat focused on pathology and may not document notable areas of strength. Testing may not reflect moderator variables, the influence of such factors as education or social and economic status, which may have an effect upon the display of clinical syndromes or underlying personality patterns. Testing is also influenced by motivational variables and context, which may influence test-taking attitude and completeness of report. With the increasing use of automated tests, it is especially important to use them to provide diagnostic direction but not diagnostic conclusions. They seem to ring more true than is justified by research or reality.

These cautions are all the more relevant in assessing depression. The general clinical tests provide only a rough measure of the presence or absence of given mood states. The MMPI, for example, has been found fairly poor in differentiating major depressive disorder from bipolar disorders, as well as in differentiating anxiety and depression (e.g., Snaith, Ahmed, Mehta, and Hamilton, 1971). The Millon inventory seems to be more effective in assessing personality disorders than Axis I clinical syndromes such as depression. Although establishing a multiaxial diagnosis is important and may be made more reliable by testing, these instruments seem exceedingly limited in terms of assessing depression

There are specific instruments designed for assessing depression. These can be divided into those that rely upon patient self-report and those which are completed by a clinician. Of the patient self-report inventories, by far the one most frequently used is the Beck Depression Inventory (BDI) (Beck, Ward, Mendelson, Mock, and Erbaugh, 1961). The original version of this test included 84 self-evaluative statements in 21 categories. The test was modified in 1971 and later copyrighted. A shorter version with 13 items correlates highly with the longer form, which is used is far more often. The

BDI measures affective (mood), cognitive, motivational, and physiological symptoms of depression. It is designed to measure depression as a singular entity and does not focus on diagnostic subtypes. The focus is on depth or severity of depressive symptoms. Hammen (1981) considers the Beck inventory the best measure among self-ratings for assessing severity of depression. A review of this instrument is provided by Beck, Steer, and Garbin (1988). It generally has good reliability and validity, as well as a very substantial history of 30 years of use, and it has figured in over 1,000 studies. Although it tends to focus on cognitive, rather than physical, signs and symptoms of depression, the BDI has been used by a number of researchers (e.g., McLean & Hakstian, 1979) to also measure response to treatment.

The Center for Epidemiological Studies has produced a depression scale (CES-D) for use in the epidemiological catchment area studies. This is a 20-item scale which measures the level of depression. Each item is rated on a four-point scale referring to the frequency of symptom presentation in the last week. An item receives a score of 0 for "no days" of presentation, with a score of 3 for 5 to 7 days of presentation. A score of 16 is recommended by the scale's author as a cutoff for diagnosing depression. There is some evidence of internal reliability and test-retest reliability (Radloff, 1977), and there are some correlations with concurrent measures (Weissman, Prusoff, and Newberry, 1975). The items include mood and physical symptoms, such as sleep and appetite disturbance, as well as emotional reactions, such as a sense of hopelessness, disproportionate guilt, or low self-worth. The CES-D is designed for use with the general population and not merely primarily in clinical studies. Lewinsohn and Teri (1982) conclude that it is better used to show those at risk for depression rather than as a diagnostic instrument.

The Zung Rating Scale for Depression (ZSRDS or SDS) is a 20-item scale designed to assess factor-analytically derived aspects of depression. Items refer to pervasive depressed mood and physiological and psychological concomitants of depression. Carroll, Fielding, and Blashki (1973) suggest that this test may not do well at differentiating different levels of depression. Zung (1965) believes that it does an adequate job of differentiating depressed from nondepressed patients.

The Multiscore Depression Inventory (MDI) (Berndt, 1986) provides a global measure of depression as well as measures on 10 subscales. Scales measure such components of depression as excessive guilt, pessimism, low self-regard, and lack of energy. The MDI includes 118 items in a forced-choice (yes-no) format. Berndt cites psychometric studies showing good internal reliability and concurrent validities as well as consistent factor studies.

Other rating scales, such as the General Health Questionnaire, Inventory to Diagnose Depression, and Inventory of Depressive Symptoms–Self-Report, have been proposed. These have not been extensively utilized nor have their reliability and validity been adequately researched.

The self-report inventories vary in their effectiveness depending upon the criterion score used. They are thought perhaps to over-report depression, by as much as two- to threefold, yielding a large number of false positives. Validating studies using the BDI report prevalence rates between two and four times the 6.8% base rate for major depressive disorder. Setting low cutoff scores, however, yields a high number of false negatives. Berndt (1990) notes that higher cutoff scores could yield an underestimation of depression for up to a third of those evaluated. Additionally, since the questionnaires measure symptoms found in both emotionally and physically based depression, no distinction between these diagnostic groups can be made.

Coulehan, Schulberg, and Block (1989) note that many of these instruments are validated by studies in which they are compared to structured interviews, the psychometric qualities of which are hardly sufficient to make them a "gold standard" for validation. As Costello (1993) so elegantly notes about structured interviews, "in passing, it is perhaps worth noting that these are peculiar validity studies in that they seem to use clinically souped up interviews to provide gold standard data against which to evaluate data from structured interviews that were initially designed to be improvements over unstructured clinical interviews" (p. 4).

Among the clinician-completed rating scales for depression, the most widely used is the Hamilton Rating Scale for Depression (Hamilton, 1968). This scale contains 20 items, of which 17 are scored by a rater during an interview. Scores range from 0 to 50, with scores of 14 or more indicating a level of depression justifying treatment, and scores of 6 or 7 generally seen as indicating remission (Ziegler, Co, Taylor, Clayton, and Biggs, 1976). The test seems to have fairly good interrated reliability and correlates quite well with other observer- and self-rating scales, suggesting concurrent validity (O'Hara and Rehm, 1983; Hedlund and Vieweg, 1979).

The Hamilton is sensitive to changes in level of depression. It has been designed to measure severity of depression and not to diagnose depression. Dunner and Schmaling (1994) suggest that it may be a better test for assessing major depressive disorder than dysthymic disorder. They note that dysthymic patients tend to score in the 16–20 point range on the Hamilton, but that mean major depression scores are in the 20–25 point range. This makes it harder to show treatment effects as a result of the lower base rate on the test and less latitude for statistical change. It has also been noted (Hellerstein, Samstag, Little, and Yanowitch, 1994) that the Hamilton tends to emphasize "vegetative" rather than "psychological" symptoms.

Other rating scales have been proposed, such as the Montgomery Asberg Depression Rating Scale (Montgomery and Asberg, 1979), Inventory of Depressive Symptomatology, Clinician rated (IDS-C) (Rush, Giles, et al., 1986), and the Bech-Rafaelson Depression Scale (BRDS) (Bech, Kastrup, and Rafaelsen, 1986). None of these have achieved the popularity and clinical reliance of the Hamilton.

These instruments measure depression once diagnosed, however, and may be better used to measure or monitor change once a multiaxial diagnosis has been made. The instruments may be better at quantifying depression than diagnosing it. One may have depressive symptoms for other reasons, such as appetite changes or weight loss as a result of delusions (for example, believing that food has been poisoned); irritability or easy fatigability can occur from a generalized anxiety disorder; sleeping problems can occur secondary to anxiety; and difficulties in concentration and attention can stem from a somatization disorder. Further, rapid changes in mood may be associated with a personality disorder, such as a borderline disorder, lack of pleasure may be found in the schizoid personality disorder, and grandiosity may be characteristic of narcissism, just as difficulty in making decisions may be due to excessive dependence.

It is important to establish a precise diagnosis for a variety of reasons relevant not only to care, but the context of care. As will be discussed, the managed care environment will emphasize specificity of treatment, documentation of diagnosis, and assessment of treatment effects. Good diagnostic data provided to the administrative level afford the opportunity for specialized system-wide interventions for differing specific conditions. Actuarial monitoring of the prevalence rates of various conditions can facilitate effective programmatic interventions.

For the clinician involved in treating a patient, monitoring treatment effects is quite important. Particularly with treatment effects from medications or other interventions, it is helpful to know if one is "on target" or not. The patient's self-report is the most often used means for measuring treatment effects. Better information is obtained by the use of rating scales, as noted earlier, or of other consistent measures of general distress, such as the Symptom Check List 90 (SCL-90) (Derogatis, Lipman, & Covi, 1973). The SCL-90 is a multidimensional self-report inventory used in over 700 research studies. This brief questionnaire takes less than 15 minutes for the patient to complete and provides both specific and global measures of symptoms and intensity. It is frequently used to consistently monitor a patient's progress in treatment.

The assessment of changes in targeted symptoms (e.g., Costello, 1993), rather than of syndromes, is a good way to proceed in evaluating treatment effects. Objective and consistent instruments are available. Given the need for strategic effort and efficient use of resources to achieve desired changes, instruments such as those discussed here may prove a helpful resource for practitioners in a managed care environment.

5

Assumptions About Treatment of Depression

The various theories, diagnoses, and understandings of depression seem very incomplete and in some cases incompatible. Correlational studies show relationships between depressive symptoms and other personal attributes for groups of people, but do little to provide information regarding the specific causes and consequences for depression with any one individual. Further, the more one considers the spectrum of research and its implications the more one becomes aware of the complexity inherent in understanding the matter.

One way to reconcile the theories discussed previously is to view the five-pointed star in Figure 1 as reflective of "points of emphasis" of individual functioning (as adapted from Corsini, 1981; Carr, 1995). A five-pointed star shares the geometric principle with the triangle that changing any one angle also causes changes in the others. In this analogy, any influence on one aspect of an individual would affect other aspects, as well. This is a way to make some sense of the complexity of individual functioning as it applies to the research on depression.

The 5-pointed star model attempts to represent a holistic view of human functioning. Holism refers to conceptualizing the "whole" as being more than merely the sum of its "parts," and the holistic view holds that people are a unity, not merely "composed of discrete parts in a clever assemblage" (Manaster and Corsini, 1982). Although Figure 1 suggests the contribution of various facets of in-

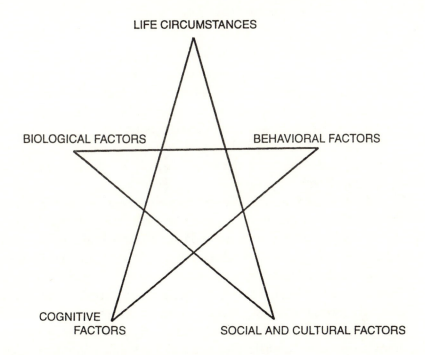

LIFE CIRCUMSTANCES

BIOLOGICAL FACTORS

BEHAVIORAL FACTORS

COGNITIVE
FACTORS

SOCIAL AND CULTURAL FACTORS

Figure 1. Interrelationship of Human Factors.

dividual functioning by something of a systems metaphor, it is also an attempt to reflect the interaction of effects in a holistic entity.

Aspects of functioning do interact. As an example, biological influences—perhaps a medical condition—may produce an entirely physiologically based disorder of mood. This might cause changes in behavior suggestive of emotional depression. For example, hypothyroidism can result in decreased physical activity, hypersomnolence, decreased libido, and decreased social activity as one's general level of activity subsides. As social activity and productive efforts diminish, social relationships are also affected, and an individual gathers fewer social rewards or reinforcements on the behavioral level. Other changes in functioning can occur, for example, loss of a job, which can affect one's role in the social network. The loss of a job and problems finding work can trigger self-disparaging thoughts on the cognitive level, and cause an individual to feel excessive guilt. Helplessness to increase one's level of motivation and activity might lead to greater pessimism about future rewards. This in turn might lead to further behavioral changes, for example, drinking or reduced physical activity, which may amplify biological dysfunction. Although the example here is of a medical rather than an emotionally based depression, it illustrates the interaction among the various focal points of individual functioning.

With emotional and behavioral conditions the same interrelationships may hold true. Robert Post, M.D. (1994), Chief of the Biological Psychiatry Branch at the National Institutes of Mental Health, speculates about how environmental events can effect physical correlates of depression. Using an example of kindling, as the theory applies to seizure activity, Post discusses how repeated cortical stimulation may not produce seizure activity until a threshold is reached after a series of recurrent stimulations, and the research animal finally has a seizure. As the seizure threshold is lowered through seizure activity, seizures occur more easily. Additionally, given the homeostasis of bodily functioning, a seizure causes the body to produce a variety of substances which allow the body to recuperate from and respond to the presence of a seizure. The body's attempt to recuperate causes other changes in the area of the brain stimulated by the seizure, much as swelling can occur as the body attempts to reinvigorate damaged muscle tissue. By analogy, Post suggests, the risk of recurrence of depression increases to the degree that it can occur more easily, even spontaneously. Post implies that a prior depression can increase later vulnerability to depression, somewhat as a previously sprained ankle is more likely to be reinjured.

The analogy may have more than illustrative validity. For example, Plotsky demonstrated that animals treated aversively in the early days of life can develop differences in a variety of limbic structures as the result. The current *zeitgeist* seems to make it easier to accept that biological aberrations can lead to psychological and behavioral deficiencies but less easy to see the converse—that biological changes can stem from psychosocial events. Interestingly, many of those having difficulty with this train of thought are also committed to physical exercise as a way to improve their physical fitness or find respite in an engrossing novel which allows them to "clear their mind" from the stresses of work and gain a sense of physical relaxation. Both research and common human experience validate the position that psychosocial therapies and events can effect physiological changes in a human organism. This view may make more understandable the research on placebo responses and even allow speculation about the sources of "error variance," those unaccounted variations of effects, in biological interventions. This does not, however, imply that psychosocial interventions are the most *efficient* way to alter system functioning when the predominant symptom display is biological.

PREDISPOSING AND PRECIPITATING FACTORS

A person can be considered as a holistic entity with specific areas of vulnerability. It is helpful to distinguish two such areas, *predisposing factors* and *precipitating factors*, in disorders of mood. Predisposing factors are those characteristics or events which place an individual more at risk for or more vulnerable to depression. Precipitating factors are "triggers" of depression present in some people. Predisposing factors can be characterized as a "weak link of the chain," while precipitating factors can be compared to an unusual load upon that weakened chain.

Predisposing factors include genetic vulnerabilities, certain anomolies of biological functioning, certain developmental traumas, and loss events. Research on disruptions in attachment or difficulties in parenting efforts after the death of a parent suggest that enduring effects can make an individual more susceptible to depression. Some skill and ability deficits may be fairly enduring, rendering an individual more vulnerable to deficiencies in social support in adult life. Disabilities or physical disfigurement might also pose a challenge in gaining a variety of rewards. Post (1994) suggests that the kindling hypothesis would apply to early and perhaps repetitive emotional traumas, lowering an individual's threshold for depression and predisposing him or her to disorders of mood.

Some personality factors can certainly constitute a predisposing factor in depression. Although there is some intriguing speculation that introversion, as used in the British sense of the term (e.g., Eysenck and Eysenck, 1968), has an innate rather than learned component, it does seem to be an enduring trait correlated with depression, as distinct from shyness (e.g., Zimbardo, 1977), which is a more learned "people avoidant strategy." Tendencies towards avoidance may also be rather enduring personality patterns, as may be excessive dependency or obsessive-compulsive behavioral patterns, all of which seem to predispose an individual to depression.

Cognitive schemas, or one's "assumptive world," may have a fairly enduring or "characterological" nature. For example, one who sees the world as filled with dangerous strangers who are best avoided may behave in socially avoidant ways and develop an interactional style which is self-fulfilling and validated by the experiences which this style of interaction creates, thus reinforcing this avoidant style of interaction. Gregory Bateson (1972) said "our lives are lived on the basis of assumptions, the validity of which is our belief in them." This is true not only in an anthropological sense. The interactional patterns from mistaken assumptions create enduring patterns of behavior which can predispose one to depression. It can be argued that personality disorders, in fact, reflect such cognitive distortions. Some consider the assumptive world to be a more available "access point" than the behavioral realm for correcting a person's "basic mistakes."

Life circumstances or cultural factors may also predispose an individual to depression. Those who are isolated or limited by situational or cultural factors are less likely to gain reward and satisfaction and thus are more vulnerable to depression. For example, males out of work are at risk for depression. Single mothers with young children, particularly those in small towns or rural environments with less opportunity for economic advancement and a smaller pool of dating eligibles, are also at greater risk.

While each of these factors might predispose an individual to depression, none would be sufficient in and of itself to *cause* depression. Some correlational studies examining depression show group differences on various dimensions which do not lead to accurate prediction on an individual level. These group studies may be measuring predisposing factors rather than precipitating ones. Distinguishing the types of factors might be one way to account for group differences. For example, this could help explain why there is increased comorbidity between twins although some people with identical biological or genetic constituencies differ in the experience of a disorder of mood: They may share predisposing factors for depression without experiencing the same precipitating events for a depressive episode. It should be recalled that even if monozygotic twins both experience a mood disorder, they may express it quite differently due to nongenetic factors.

Among the precipitating factors for depression, loss or the threat of loss in significant relationships seems important both in psychological theory and research. "Exit events," in which people experiences some loss in their lives or abrupt life changes, have been found to be such precipitating events. Symbolic losses can also be a factor. A significant birthday for an ambitious but aging businessman may redefine his view of self and serve as a signal for the need to limit aspirations. For the recently bereaved woman attempting to resurrect closeness, a singles' dance attended only by other single widows might be the "straw that breaks the camel's back" if she is particularly vulnerable to depressive episodes.

Changes in social support or social role may precipitate depression. Holmes and Rahe (1967) suggest that life changes, whether good or bad, can produce significant negative psychological and physical effects. These life changes can certainly correlate with differences in level of social support, just as inheriting a fortune and quitting work would result in a loss of social contact at a job to the same degree as being fired, even though wealth might make it easier to gain other satisfactions.

New developmental tasks or challenges can certainly be a precipitating stress. Graduating from school, getting married, the birth of a child, divorce, widowhood, a move to a new city, a new job, or a promotion at work can all demand new coping skills and constitute a stress. Certain physical events, such as lack of sleep, changes in level of exercise, and even dietary changes, which in some serve as transitory stresses or prompt brief moments of demoralized mood, constitute a profound discouragement for others, accumulating to prompt a depressive reaction.

METHODS FOR INTERVENTION

A holistic view facilitates a focus on different aspects of the functioning of an integrated and indivisible human entity. Not only can predisposing and precipitating factors be asigned to different points on the star in Figure 1, but interventions can also cluster around these focal points. Biological interventions constitute one category of therapeutic efforts and include use of medicines, light therapy, intentional changes in sleep patterns, and increases in physical activity.

Behavioral changes can be achieved by such interventions as coping skills classes. For example, interventions targeting social withdrawal might range from classes on "flirting" and engaging others in social interactions to programs in "overcoming shyness" to assertiveness training. Monitoring pleasurable events and increasing the rate of contingency-based reward are examples of behavioral interventions which can reverberate throughout the human system.

Cognitive changes can occur through a variety of cognitive and behavioral approaches. These might be based on Beck's cognitive behavior therapy, Adler's lifestyle analysis, Kelly's role construct theory, or any of the efforts directed at changing attributional styles, particularly relevant with some who are experiencing depression. Cognitive interventions may be enhanced by a variety of behavioral interventions or vice versa.

Traditional therapy has often focused on changing the individual's personality and ability to react to stress. In managed care, therapy will also likely focus upon changing one's circumstances, looking at ways that one might increase reinforcement availability, or overcoming change events by developing alternative rewards or transitional support. Examples include looking at new ways to meet people through developing different activities or pursuits, considering changing a job for which a person is now ill suited, and exploring vocational guidance or financial counseling to help with changes in employment status. Marital and family intervention, either through therapy or guided education, may lead to positive environmental or life change, which can be particularly effective with those whose marital problems seem a pronounced precipitant for depression.

Social and cultural factors contributing to depression can be addressed through counseling which focuses upon revisiting major life decisions of vocational choice or commitment to certain values or pursuits, or upon reunderstanding a dilemma and making a choice to persist with a way of life. An element of control and mastery might be added by defining as intentional the decision to stay in a small town, to persist with a family farm, to remain a vocal member of an unpopular religious minority, or to view unalterable social change in broader perspective.

Focusing on social and cultural factors might also allow a sufficiently large managed care program to develop interventions to reduce the risk of psychological problems for certain classes of individuals. A large program could, for example, provide mentoring programs for young single mothers by volunteer grandmothers or respite care for those with aging parents. Such efforts can be efficient and measurable in their success in achieving targeted changes for specified groups of individuals at risk for depression.

NEED FOR A THEORY

Managed care efforts necessitate some consistency of theory and treatment approach, as does perhaps any effective attempt to help another (see, for example, Frank, 1973). Theory gives direction and focus. The therapist needs to know what to ignore as well as what to treat. The question becomes which theory to adopt, and when to adopt it, not whether a theory is necessary.

George Kelly (1955) proposed what might be viewed as a cognitive theory of personality and therapy. In discussing the application of theories to different situations he suggests that theories have a scope of convenience as well as a scope of utility. He considered the *focus of convenience* of a theory the area for which a theory or method is particularly well suited. The *range of applicability* is the total domain in which the theory or method can be applied.

It appears that any one of the competing theories, be it psychological, sociocultural, or biological, could be applied to any one of the depressive disorders, since each theory has a *range of applicability* that covers all of the disorders of mood. Some theories, however, are most applicable for certain ranges of conditions and others have very limited utility or potency for guiding treatment of some conditions. In short, their foci of convenience differ. Viewing theories in this way can allow a provider to choose a "functional fit" for a specific patient with a specific set of symptoms, rather than to take a rigid and invariant approach to treatment.

There are a variety of ways to look at the various depressive conditions. One can sort disorders of mood along the dimension of the more to the less biologically involved. This continuum might also reflect the less to the more psychosocially involved nature of the different depressive conditions. While there are problems in a holistic view in overemphasizing such a conceptual dichotomy between biological and psychosocial factors, the depressive conditions do seem to vary regarding the presence and importance of physical symptomatology and the involvement of biological shifts and genetic contributions. This spectrum is even enforced by the nomenclature that lists changes in sleep, appetite, and weight among the diagnostic criteria for bipolar and major depressive disorders, for example. Other disorders, such as those associated with grief reactions, dysthymia, or problems with bereavement, have more behavioral or mood-based diagnostic criteria. Figure 2 illustrates one way in which these conditions could be categorized according to the contribution or significance of biological factors in a depressive syndrome.

Simultaneously, this diagram illustrates the relative likely contribution of psychosocial factors to the signs and symptoms within a diagnostic condition. Since comparatively more of the contribution would be caused by biological factors at one end of the continuum, and more by psychosocial factors at the other, it seems that some conditions are more "medical" in their nature and others more "psychological." This would suggest that medical consultation and the prescription of psychotropic medicines, for example, would be more indicated toward the left side of the continuum, for bipolar or major depressive disorders, but less likely to be helpful for the more "characterological" depressions on the right side of the continuum, those which seem to play a functional role within a distressed family system, or that reflect difficulties in adjusting to transitions in life or deficits in coping skills. This also implies the psychological interventions that stem from psychological theories are less likely to be

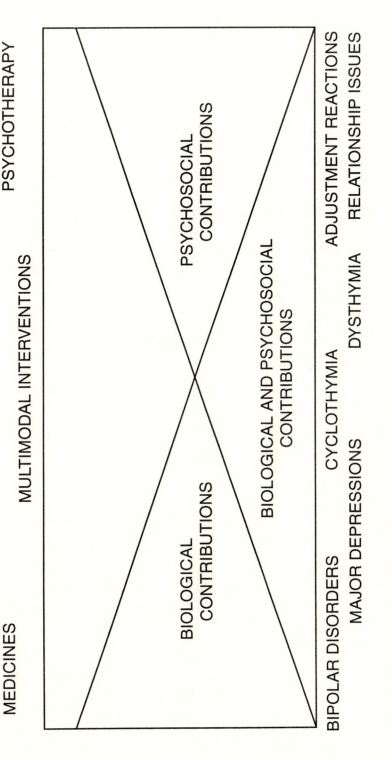

Figure 2. Conditions and Interventions.

efficient as treatment for conditions which arise more from biological factors. There is a *focus of convenience* for more psychologically focused theories on the right end of the continuum, and a *focus of convenience* for biological factors on the left. Psychological and biological approaches might equally have wide ranges of applicability and serve as a possible treatment approach for perhaps 80 to 90% of the spectrum of mood disorders, but certain approaches would be *best suited* for certain disorders.

NEED TO UNDERSTAND SOCIAL CONTEXT

In addition to adopting a holistic view of human functioning and encouraging flexibility, the authors also strongly advocate attempting to understand an individual within a social context. This is illustrated by Figure 3. An individual exists and operates on a variety of different levels simultaneously. Understanding a person at only one level of functioning is very limiting and therapeutically very inefficient.

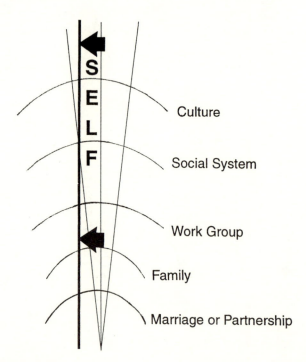

Figure 3. Function and Balance.

It is culture and context that provide meaning to human experience. Cultural values, social meaning, and a shared language of custom, norm, and action are essential aspects of understanding a person. It is only through appreciating the many levels within which a person operates–the social field or context–that a therapist can adequately understand and therefore effectively help the patient. The social psychological and cultural context give the patient's "story" its meaning. Our view is that people exist only within a social context. Decontextualizing an individual, seeing symptoms as separate from the social milieu, seeing an individual as unrelated to his or her social world, or viewing a system as independent of human experience and meaning, is to "miss the mark" of understanding and treating psychopathology (see, for example, Kleinman and Good, 1985).

A person's simultaneous and effective functioning in a variety of social contexts is illustrated in Figure 3. The "alignment" of an individual within these various contexts produces harmony, social reward, satisfaction, and perhaps happiness. Much as a key opens a lock by aligning each of the tumblers within, so, too, does the "personal fit" between self and collective interpersonal demands on a variety of levels depend on multiple alignment. A change at any one level reverberates through the others.

As Karl Jaspers (1968) has pointed out, there is a difference between understanding and explaining. We need to "understand" as well as "explain" our patients, or at least to "explain" them more completely. Some have proposed that there is a dichotomy between understanding a person's phenomenological and contextual "story," on the one hand, and understanding him or her as a biological or objectified "separate" organism, on the other (e.g., Verhulst, 1995). We believe that appreciating the context within which a person lives allows a depth of understanding which would otherwise be lacking. Effective interventions, appropriately specialized and targeted goals, and enduring benefits from treatment will not occur without understanding patients within their social contexts.

There is an additional reason to attend to contextual issues. Figure 4 is an attempt to illustrate the effects on an individual who is in disharmony or fails to blend in with the demands of different levels of social contexts, one who is "off center" or imbalanced. In our

view this reflects both social and psychological dysfunction. A review of diagnostic nomenclature, such as in *DSM-IV*, reveals that
the diagnoses ultimately reflect ways in which an individual is dys-
functional both psychiatrically *and* in terms of social functioning.
An individual who is able to work and love, using Freud's standards, or achieve the goals of work, love, and community, using
Adler's basic challenges, would not receive any psychiatric diagnosis.

We also believe that individual functioning affects others and is
affected by others. Effectively responding to a person takes into
account both the social causes and consequences in the human system and the interaction between the individual and social context.
It truly is a dance. To be effective the therapist must be aware that
the patient is dancing in a unique social ballroom, lest he or she
step on the patient's feet inadvertently. This also implies that therapy,
however best indicated, would ultimately be focused upon helping
an individual achieve some measure of not only psychological, but
also psychosocial harmony.

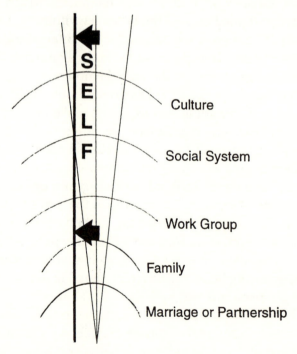

Figure 4. Dysfunction and Imbalance.

SUMMARY

Regardless of the greater applicability of some theories than others to certain conditions, some flexibility of approach seems warranted even for those who share similar diagnoses. The authors appreciate the need for a range of interventions for a range of problems and call for flexibility throughout the creative process of treatment. This flexibility is even more essential in a managed care context, where appropriateness of therapeutic efforts is necessitated by the limited nature of resources. Regardless of what specific theory or intervention is deemed appropriate to a problem or patient, the authors advocate a continuing appreciation for the holistic nature of human functioning within a social context. We see any theory as limited which singles out aspects of individual functioning. Although it is necessary to segregate variables for treatment or research in specific contexts, people should be treated as singular entities, not as unrelated biological components and psychosocial components. While the term "holism" may conjure up faddish therapies of years gone by, there is a philosophical justification (e.g., Smuts, 1961; Adler, 1966) and research support for a holistic view of functioning in which an individual's complexity and depth are appreciated.

6

Treatment of Depression in the New Ecology

The context of treatment in managed care converges with the theoretical understandings of depression to produce a treatment approach. Although some argue that protocol-based interventions for specific syndromes are warranted, the more viable approach considers *principles* of treatment suited for a treatment context rather than to specify treatment practices or to attempt to develop universally valid protocol-based interventions. A helpful way to develop such principles of treatment is to review the "six d's" of treatment in managed care as they apply to treatment of depression. We believe that treatment in managed care will be: *diagnostic, directive, delegated, didactic, documented,* and *delimited.*

DIAGNOSTIC TREATMENT

There is a need for clinical *diagnosis,* almost certainly involving a multiaxial method such as described in the *DSM.* This is necessary for resource utilization and management and research. A reliable diagnosis will be necessary for developing a treatment plan, to allow authorization for treatment, and for treatment review. Although diagnostically related groupings of patients have generally been applied only to determine reimbursement for ongoing care on an inpatient basis, it is certainly possible that diagnoses will determine the length of outpatient treatment authorized. One can imagine, for example, an authorization for six sessions for the diagnosis of an adjustment reaction with depression, 10 sessions for major depressive disorders and 14 sessions for dysthymic disorder.

Although this book focuses on individual treatment of depression, it should be remembered that managed care is collective care offered to groups of enrolled members. This necessitates monitoring utilization and gathering epidemiological data within these groups. More sophisticated managed care programs which provide mental health services to a large number of people will need group approaches for the high percentage of people diagnosed as having any particular problem. Correlations between rates of medical utilization and the use of treatment for various Axis I conditions would be a helpful way to gauge the system-wide economic benefit of mental health services. Such research will require precision of diagnosis.

Diagnosis needs to go further, however, for the clinician providing services in managed care. While depression is certainly a focal syndrome, the diagnostic nomenclature indicates some differences in types of depression and even allows for variability of sign and symptom display among those with the same diagnosis. Targeting and measuring changes in specific signs will facilitate the monitoring of various intervention effects. This information helps the clinician and provides indicators of quality assurance to the external reviewer. As an example, major depressive disorder can include a host of specific symptoms, such as frequent suicidal thoughts, physical difficulties, social withdrawal, impaired information processing, and faulty cognitive functioning. Physical symptoms might be broken down into specific problems of insomnia, physical slowing, and significant weight or appetite reduction. Each of these symptoms is amenable to assessment and monitoring. There is likely to be an increasing emphasis on specificity in the managed care setting, according to Goldfried and Castonguay (1992) and Strupp (1992), among others.

Monitoring of improvement will also have to be more rigorous in a managed care context, both to ensure therapeutic outcome and for quality assurance assessment. Global measures of improvement, based on asking patients how they feel or on observations made during the therapy hour, will likely be replaced by more objective ratings, standardized assessment of improvement in targeted dimensions, and reference to consistent measurement devices. It is one thing, for example, for a patient to say, "I'm not sure these pills are helping," and another to note a five-point improvement on the Hamilton Depression Inventory over a course of five weeks on an antidepressant medicine. In the same way, inquiries about mood may produce vaguer results than measures of improvement in appetite, of productivity at work, or a spouse's reports about improvements in sleep or reductions in drinking.

It is also important in diagnosis to attend to other factors relevant to treatment. As we proposed in Chapter 5, decontextualizing an individual and evaluating signs, symptoms, and clinical conditions without understanding the person is a very limited and mechanical way to approach personal problems. This approach provides knowledge but not meaning, information but not understanding.

Such factors as personal resources are certainly a component to care and are important in treatment planning. A depressed single mother in a low-income job is at high risk for depression. The limitations on her time and financial resources must be taken into account if a treatment plan is to be effective. One's intellectual level and educational resources are also important. Handouts about depression and social activity will hardly be meaningful to a seclusive, private person who is semiliterate. Treatment in which the therapist uses very abstract metaphors and analogies may "miss the mark" for someone with an IQ of 82.

The social supports available to an individual should be evaluated. The presence or absence of family dysfunction or of a supportive spouse is clearly relevant as a correlate of depression and somewhat predictive of success of treatment. Awareness of these factors might, at a minimum, lead to considering involving a spouse in treatment or providing diagnostic or treatment information to the family. Such knowledge also affects treatment. For example, one who has recently moved to a new city and works in an isolated situation would be hard-pressed to quickly implement advice to increase his or her level of social interaction unless that person had remarkable social skills. The therapist should suggest other options.

Knowing not only the presence but the depth of such support is important. Someone with more enduring relationships has a greater reservoir of social support than the person who has more superficial social support or whose social support is contingent upon stature, appearance, or acquiescence. The therapist would need to assess these relevant aspects to a patient's circumstances.

Finally, some assessment and appreciation of the patient's social ecology seems to be a vital aspect of diagnosing not only the condition but the life of the person who displays that condition. Since people exist simultaneously within a number of systems and subsystems, an effective intervention takes into account the effects of change on each of those systems. Increased assertiveness may be a very valid intervention, but even an effective assertiveness class and the patient's demonstration of behavioral skills of assertiveness may not guarantee success without attention to the individual's social ecology. For example, a rigidly religious, highly traditional, and socially unsophisticated family may consider the wife's appropriate role to be that of submission to the husband's authority. A change in level of assertiveness without acknowledging the influence of this social context might be ineffective and could even intensify marital discord. Involving the husband in the wife's treatment, perhaps offering information about assertiveness to the spouse, or even involving the spouse in a teaching role might preserve the *structure* of the relationship and allow appropriate behavioral changes on an individual level.

As further examples, recommending sedating tricylic antidepressants to facilitate sleep onset and continuity might not be helpful for the mother who needs to attend to a young child whose asthmatic symptoms occasionally become worse at night. Recommending an increase in mirth and levity as a way to enhance one's interpersonal desirability might backfire if the client is a judge or a minister for whom the small town public may hold very rigid expectations of role-governed behavior. Stressing increased independence from parents might intensify role conflicts with a first-generation Asian American whose cultural heritage values a more committed response to elders.

Diagnosis is important in managed care for a variety of reasons. Diagnosis must make use of a common vernacular, as exemplified in the *DSM* diagnostic nomenclature. It must be specific about symptoms, but broad about the person who displays them. It must be useful to those outside the treatment context, such as managers and auditors, but also allow treatment which will ultimately help an individual totally separate from such managerial concerns.

DIRECTIVE TREATMENT

Treatment in managed care will certainly need to be *directive*. The therapist will have to play an active role in leading, guiding, directing, and developing alternatives. Goals for treatment must be defined in a treatment plan. As is sometimes said, "If you don't know where you're going, you will end up somewhere else." This, too, is true for therapy. Managed care implies direction of goal with efficient steps taken to reach those goals. There is little latitude for meandering, and the context is designed to meet only certain delimited and authorized goals.

A metaphor for managed care might be that of shopping. Some view shopping as a process, saying things such as "I think I'll go shopping today." Some people enjoy going through the mall and finding a host of creative ideas for decorating or dining, browsing in new stores, and perhaps finding better values over the course of the day. A person may start off with a general interest in clothing, but return from the mall with a preparation for fondue. Shopping in this case is something of an end in itself, an activity which can be deemed successful even if one returns empty-handed, given the enjoyment of the occasion and the pleasurable nature of this activity for some people.

Shopping in a world of managed care is much different. Here, the therapist is given a quite specific shopping list, with limited time to accomplish it. A managed care therapist is assumed to know where the best values can be had and will choose the store based on prices rather than on friendship with the shopkeeper. "Shopping" will be a task to be accomplished, so that the managed care therapist can move on to the next assignment. The managed care therapist who returns from a day's activity and enthusiastically reports that nothing from the list was purchased, but that the shopping was enjoyable, or that other good purchases were made instead, will not be viewed favorably by the managed care agencies and may not be sent on further shopping missions.

To pursue the analogy even further, one may assume that the managed care agencies will vary in terms of the specificity of items on the shopping list. Some companies might authorize the therapist to go to the store and purchase all the ingredients for a reasonably priced dinner for a family of four. This company might assume that the therapist has some knowledge of nutrition, value, and tastes in his or her area. Good alternatives could range from pasta to fish for a main dish, with a wide array of vegetable and bread accompaniments. This approach allows the therapist room for creative involvement, resulting in a meal more likely to meet the needs of a family or a specific context.

Another managed care company may be quite specific, stipulating, for example, that the therapist should provide a dinner for four composed of specific ingredients of vegetables, spices, proportions, and so on, to be cooked at a certain time. This approach makes the therapist less a director than an errand person.

Such an approach seems ill-advised. If the therapist is selected from those competent to make appropriate choices, he or she is in a better situation to know what vegetables are in season and a particular family's preferences for highly seasoned foods versus more bland ones. The therapist would know that the food needs to cook longer in Colorado, for example, than in San Diego, since higher elevations cause water to boil at slightly lower temperatures and affect the length of simmering necessary.

The managed care therapist will need to be assertive and directive not only with the patient, but also by communicating in cooperative and goal-consonant ways with the managed care organization. If it is true that managed care companies are authentically concerned with achieving therapeutic goals, cooperative communication of this kind is quite important. The managed care therapist needs to direct effective change for the patient, but may also need to provide guidance and direction for the managed care company, as well. This can be done in a spirit of mutual respect. There is little cause to assume managed care companies to be ill motivated when they may merely be uninformed.

There is a difference between being directive and being dictatorial. Directive forms of treatment, particularly in time-limited treatment, demand patient cooperation. The therapist in such a context must contend with limitations of resources and time and, frankly, can use all the help he or she can get. Alliance with the patient is vital to meeting this challenge. Nonresponsive or inflexible approaches are likely to be counterproductive. The theme should be activity and direction toward goals, not condescension or domination.

The therapist may be viewed as a leader in a team of equals, even if that team is comprised of only the therapist and the patient. Treatment must be viewed as a mutual endeavor, with the therapist seen as a normal human being with specialized knowledge and specific expertise. Any other form of relationship could impede the flow of communication that is necessary for developing valid treatment goals, refining them based on feedback, accurately measuring outcomes, and ensuring use of services and access to future care by the patient, after a good initial experience.

Similarly, the managed care therapist needs to focus on goals in a human context and not take too literally the metaphor of therapist as mechanic. Depression occurs in people, not in machines, and the therapist must have a personal relationship with the patient in order for therapy to be effective. Therapy can still be a rewarding and personal experience for both therapist and client, with opportunities for rapport and an appreciation of the narrative aspects as well as the mechanical and medical sides of a patient's symptom picture. One needs to understand "the story" and truly know the patient, but in a context that encourages getting specific things done quickly.

DELEGATED TREATMENT

Managed care requires that therapeutic tasks be accomplished in order to achieve therapeutic goals, but that does not mean that the therapist is charged with accomplishing those goals in the therapy session. In fact, it would be quite difficult and certainly inefficient to attempt to accomplish therapeutic goals only through the vehicle of therapy. Viewing therapeutic change as involving a variety of components allows an appraisal of which vehicles or mechanisms are best to achieve desired outcomes. There are far more efficient and effective ways than psychotherapy to achieve some objectives in the treatment plan.

For example, on the assumption that relaxation techniques would be helpful at some point in treatment, the therapist might instruct the patient in this behavioral skill through one of the many available relaxation protocols. The therapist can take two sessions to teach relaxation training, monitor progress in the course of later sessions, and inquire about benefits from time to time. Casual follow-up might lead to a low-to-moderate level of continuing practice of relaxation exercises on the part of the patient. A realistic expectation might be that one out of three patients will practice exercises to the point of receiving benefit. The cost would be two therapist hours of productivity, a high level of manpower involvement, and a low level of efficiency.

A more efficient approach might be structured classes which meet for three weeks and instruct 10 people in relaxation techniques. Follow-up with a weekly five-minute phone call to each patient for two weeks might afford significantly higher levels of compliance, with perhaps as many as one half to two thirds of patients continuing to practice or participate in such interventions. The class could be run by an educational technician, who could have a less expensive level of expertise than that of a therapist at the doctoral level or a master's level. Multimodal educational techniques could be used, such as videotapes, charts, diagrams, and audiotaped practice procedures, increasing the effectiveness of these efforts. A group context might also achieve simultaneous objectives, such as increasing the rate of social interaction for depressed patients. A spouse could be inexpensively involved, perhaps contributing to a treatment approach for depression which emphasizes problem solving by the family or allows some generalization of benefit to others in the family system who are also distressed.

In addition to these additional possible benefits of treatment, such a program would be efficient. The total time required, even assuming a ten-hour program, including time for charting, follow-up, and communication with the primary therapeutic coordinator, could be less than ten hours for a total "class session." The total cost–benefit ratio, given ten hours of a therapist's time and ten people more effectively treated, would even be less, half as much on a per-hour basis, given one hour devoted to each patient. If one considers the possible use of less expensive staff resources, the cost savings for the plan and patient are even greater. Serendipitous benefits might occur in this therapeutic program which are more likely to achieve designated therapeutic objectives.

Community resources can be utilized in a course of treatment directed by the therapist who sees the goal as coordinating care, often delegating it, rather than providing it personally. Community colleges often provide excellent programs for vocational guidance and consultation. Anger management programs available through women's centers or domestic violence programs can be a helpful component to treatment for depression in those whose behavior complicates their personal relationships. Self-help programs for the dually diagnosed patient, assertiveness training classes, and parenting classes are examples of community-based programs that can promote patient skill development and reduce significant life stress.

If one views developmental stages as producing changes in one's life that demand new coping skills, be they attitudinal or behavioral, acquisition of these skills can certainly help with both treating and preventing the recurrence of depression. Parenting classes may equip a young parent with greater knowledge and therefore more efficacy to deal with typical problems of newborns. Financial management training and credit counseling resources can help those whose careers have changed to deal with such transitions in a more deliberate manner. Postdivorce educational or support groups can be helpful, as can programs targeted to help those whose spouses have died, to become emotionally and economically more self-sufficient.

Programs and activities available to the public, which were designed for other purposes, may also have therapeutic value. Exercises classes, bicycling clubs, hiking clubs, public speaking clubs, music societies, and voluntary and charitable organizations may be therapeutic resources. If the goal is to increase physical activity, exercise or physical recreation programs can provide a context and structure making a patient's exercise more regular and perhaps even socially more rewarding. If the goal is to increase social activity, a shared task among like-minded people at a volunteer organization might be an excellent vehicle. If the goal is to diversify one's "emotional portfolio" by finding rewards and satisfactions away from work or family, hobby groups may provide both social reinforcement and interesting diversions. For example, Toastmasters is an organization designed to further one's ability to speak in the public arena. It also provides a way for people with some social hesitancy to develop greater skillfulness and social comfort. Even bowling leagues can provide an opportunity for regular relaxation and comradeship that can be helpful for the overly diligent or overextended person.

The "treatment team" may be very large indeed, perhaps involving community resources, educational resources, as well as resources that are specifically designed to be therapeutic. The message of therapy in managed care is that therapeutic outcomes need to be achieved by the most effective means possible. Therapy may ultimately be more useful if it is construed as coordinating rather than providing therapeutic changes. Creativity and a knowledge of the community can certainly enable the therapist to meet a patient's needs more effectively.

Of course, this philosophy of utilizing available resources also generalizes to more formal members of the treatment team. The physician on the primary medical care level can be an important treatment ally. As noted, most psychotropic medicines are prescribed on the primary care level, and not on a psychiatric level. A relationship with a general internist, family physician, or other specialist providing primary medical care to a patient is important for coordinating care. As will be discussed below, not all depressive disorders which respond to medication necessarily require the expense of limited and valuable psychiatric resources. Assuming an accurate diagnosis on the psychological level and a thorough understanding of the patient's medical status on the primary medical care level, coordinated efforts and treatment with psychotropic medicines of the more "routine" depressive problems can occur on the primary medical care level, as demonstrated by the work of Katon et al. (1995).

The primary care physician may also be an excellent resource for information about the patient's history of compliance with other medical interventions, the likelihood of underreported alcohol or substance misuse problems, or information that the patient may not have provided or the therapist may not have collected. Such information as significant stress with a parent's terminal illness or a spouse's recurrent sexually transmitted diseases is quite helpful in providing appropriate and effective care. It is plain that the physician is an important component of the therapeutic treatment team.

It also deserves note that group therapy will almost certainly play a large role in the managed care context. Although group treatment is beyond the scope of this book, it should be acknowledged that the general diagnostic and treatment principles discussed so far are equally applicable in a group context as in an individual one. Depending upon one's view of the role of the therapist, individual and group treatment can certainly proceed simultaneously. One should not be adverse to delegating certain parts of the therapeutic endeavor to the group therapist, and the therapist should be clear about those situations in which group treatment has clear advantages, both in terms of outcome and economic efficiency.

Finally, much can be delegated to the patient. Self-help programs, behavioral programs, general goals for which the patient is encouraged to develop behavioral change protocols, and behavioral monitoring are all parts of the treatment process. Treatment is cooperative, even though directive, in the managed care context. The patient must play a role in a mutual endeavor of achieving therapeutic goals. Therapy cannot be viewed as a "gift" that a therapist provides a patient.

DIDACTIC TREATMENT

Treatment in the managed care context is often *didactic*. Although many forms of treatment may be experiential and emotive, it is hard to imagine a very focused and time-limited form of treatment that does not involve some cognitive understanding, on the part of both therapist and patient, of what is occurring. It is almost imperative that a patient understands what is happening and participates in treatment planning in order to have a more pleasant life as an outcome. An intellectual understanding of this process seems essential. This can be accomplished with respect for the patient's capacity to understand.

Depression can be explained to patients through the use of analogy and metaphor that can translate more abstract understandings into those more meaningful to the patient. For example, the primary author has found it helpful to compare depression to a stereo or balancing scale, with one channel of the stereo or one side of the scale representing the hassles, effort, and negative aspects of any activity or endeavor. The right channel, or the other side of the balance, represents the rewards or replenishments. Characteristically, the rewards outweigh the negative side, and people feel fulfilled.

To illustrate the metaphor, consider going to a movie. This activity presents the burdens and "aversive events" of driving to the theater, parking the car, waiting in line, paying for the ticket, sitting in chairs not as comfortable as those at home, and listening as people talk, cough, or drop popcorn boxes throughout the movie. The movie, however, or perhaps the social experience, makes it all seem worthwhile. After a good movie, one leaves feeling invigorated and glad to have gone.

With the depressed patient, however, the capacity to experience pleasure is diminished, as if the right channel on the stereo were turned down. To them it is like seeing a 15-minute movie. When asked if the acting was good, they'll agree. When asked about the screenplay and cinematography, they will admit to their intricacy and beauty. When asked if they want to go again next week, they will decline, largely because the ride is not worth the fare.

We have had much luck in having people accept a metaphor like this as a way to introduce the planning of behavioral or biochemical changes that can make rewards available again. In talking about medicines, for example, the metaphor can be invoked by explaining that they help the movies last their true length though do not necessarily make them good. It is up to the person to choose "movies" selectively, but the medicines may afford them an opportunity to experience pleasure if something pleasurable occurs. Many find this to be a helpful way to view their situation and a good way to distinguish antidepressants from euphoricants, or "happy pills."

Explaining the difference between depression and unhappiness can be done in a number of ways. With the more formal and medically focused patient, comparing depressive reactions (or other psychological problems) to blood pressure might be in order. It can be explained that blood pressure increases in response to certain situations, such as exercise. It is supposed to. After one finishes exercising and a period of time goes by, the blood pressure tends to subside. It only requires treatment when it goes up and stays up, regardless of the current situation. This analogy can sometimes be helpful in explaining the distinction between depression and grief.

Helping patients understand the distinction between depression and unhappiness may also be helpful in treatment. A metaphor sometimes used in this regard is that of the 58-year-old man whose wife is on dialysis, who was recently laid off from his job, and who is losing his health insurance. This person may feel terribly defeated after applying for jobs and finding himself unable to obtain work, feeling hopeless, and having a sense of despair, even failure, at the inability to provide for his loved one. Then, walking home at night though the cold, gray evening, this man chances upon a lottery ticket left on the street, and picking it up and out of curiosity taking it in for redemption, discovers it to be a big winner. That man would be happy. The depressed person, experiencing less drastic circumstances and winning the lottery, might be more inclined to say "Damn! There goes my privacy!"

The use of metaphorical communications can make more complex relationships or events very understandable to patients. Although specific personal styles or different relationships between therapist and patient may suggest a need for different communication styles, it certainly is desirable to make one's professional knowledge available to patients in ways that are meaningful for them. Didactic information about the nature of a syndrome, what causes it, and what can be mutually planned to overcome it is an essential part of managed care.

Resources are available to aid in this endeavor, such as the videotapes of New Harbinger Publications, and books, such as *Feeling Good* by David Burns (1980) and *Control Your Depression* by Lewinsohn, Muñoz, Youngren, and Zeiss (1986). Handouts are available which explain depression. *Depression, A Treatable Illness: A*

Patient's Guide is highly recommended and is provided for free by the Department of Health and Human Services Agency for Health Care Policy and Research (April, 1993). The Depression Awareness Recognition and Treatment (DART) Program also provides free publications about depression for persons of all ages, including adolescents and the aging. Books and pamphlets can also be obtained through the National Alliance for the Mentally Ill, National Depressive and Manic Depressive Association, the National Foundation for Depressive Illness, and the National Mental Health Association. These resources can add an aura of credibility to treatment and can also reinforce the idea that depression is a solvable problem, one experienced by others. This can reassure patients that their problems do not make them different from others.

Bibliotherapy can be a powerful component to treatment (see Wollersheim & Wilson, 1991; Quackenbush, 1991; Scogin, Jamison, and Davis, 1990; Ellis, 1993). Within the past half decade, over 300 new references have been listed in the professional literature about bibliotherapy. Such didactic interventions seem encouraged by changing shifts in health care. Their value is now being validated and appreciated.

Self-help and bibliotherapy are very popular among the public and are endorsed by the majority of professionals. Starker (1988) found that more than 85% of psychologists in one study found such books helpful and almost two thirds encouraged their clients to read them. Although some (e.g., Rosen 1993) point out possible disadvantages to self-help books and cassettes, many of these disadvantages can be minimized if self-help techniques are integrated into therapy, directed by the therapist, and used as one of a variety of interventions to alter targeted behavior. It serves the problem-focused therapist well to be aware of some of the popular literature that may be relevant to a range of client problems.

Didactic information on medicines is particularly helpful. As will be discussed more extensively, better compliance almost invariably occurs with patients who are better informed and who participate in the decision to use medicines. Not only is compliance more likely to occur, but the risk of serious side effects, drug misuse, and drug and alcohol interactions is reduced for the patient who understands the risks and benefits of such medicines. Unrealistic expectations can result in discontinuance of medicine or even of treatment. Understanding alternatives to use of medicines and the actions of medicines may help a patient develop realistic expectations of their effect.

The use of technology in providing information is available to those who wish to use education as a component of treatment. Videotaped explanations for medicine effects can ensure a consistent message to patients, not only providing a more reliable means of educational transmission, but also promoting compliance with legal informed-consent standards through the use of consistent and verifiable messages. Since research suggests that a single oral presentation may have limited value, redundant or supplemental efforts, such as handouts, tapes, and verbal explanations, are certainly appropriate. The managed care environment would encourage such didactic interventions to enhance patient understanding since they are generally efficient and often very helpful.

DOCUMENTED TREATMENT

Treatment in managed care will have to be documented. Documentation will afford communication with the variety of audiences who will need information in the team-treatment approach that managed care requires. Communication with managers will also necessitate documentation of diagnosis, treatment plan, and perhaps interventions. Such information is essential to effective management and utilization of resources. Quality assurance standards will depend on documentation of diagnosis and interventions, and perhaps the monitoring of steps towards therapeutic goals and treatment outcomes.

Team approaches to treatment cannot occur without some coordination of information. Information must flow between the primary therapist and the primary physician, between the individual therapist and the group therapist, and perhaps even between a primary therapist making a referral and the person providing skills training in specific areas. Documentation of both treatment efforts and results is important. Particularly with a condition such as depression, which is likely to be recurrent, the comparative effectiveness or ineffectiveness of various treatment alternatives needs to be documented. With managed care one is often providing services to a population over time, rather than merely treating a single episode. Providers will ultimately be reimbursed for outcomes, not units of service, and the outcomes in the more sophisticated systems will focus on reducing future risks as well as on current treatment needs. Enhancing the overall emotional health of a defined group will be the goal. Documentation facilitates informed and coordinated efforts to achieve this goal.

As therapists are increasingly seen as information specialists, they will need to use technology to communicate information efficiently. Managed care will almost invariably occur in a group context. Even though those groups may not be geographically proximate or physically connected, they are likely to be connected through information networks. A database of a patient's needs and system responses and resources will almost certainly be kept, both on an individual and a whole-group basis. Some knowledge of computer technology and of the ways to transmit information other than by the printed word will certainly be important. Practitioners will have to make accommodations to networked database and word processing formats. Standard protocols for information dissemination and review will promote efficiency within a managed care context and are almost certain to evolve.

The need for team approaches to personal problems necessitates access to personal information but also imposes a challenge to privacy. Historically the therapist–patient relationship was seen as akin to the confessional—secret, private, and sacrosanct, kept separate and away from other eyes. Privacy has been important, and ethical codes of all of the mental health professions require some acknowledgment of a patient's right to privacy. Even the Hippocratic Oath refers to the need to keep information gained in the course of treatment private and secret. Ethical codes of the American Psychological Association and other professions articulate similar standards for maintaining patient confidence. This seems to conflict with the free sharing of information about a patient within a treatment team.

Several accommodations need to be made to protect confidentiality and privacy. First, patient information must be kept *within the treatment context*. Information necessary for the delivery of services must be protected institutionally to the same standard as formerly afforded by an individual provider. In other words, there must be some institutional promise of confidentiality although various participants may provide collective treatment in a managed care context.

Second, the individual provider must be attentive to the needs for information on the part of the recipient and must limit extraneous information in order to provide some reassurance for privacy. There is a difference between what is relevant to "understanding" the narrative story of the patient and what is necessary for communicating a diagnosis and treatment plan. For example, a claims review specialist in a managed care situation needs to understand that a patient has experienced a major depressive reaction for the first time, that it was apparently precipitated by pronounced stress within the family, and that displayed symptoms include sleep discontinuity, weight loss of 15 pounds in 6 weeks, decreased productivity, social avoidance, depressed mood, and pessimism. It is not relevant for the claims manager to understand that the patient became depressed after finding his wife involved with a parish priest, a sexual liaison that had lasted for some years, that he feels a sense of tremendous betrayal by both church and family, and that he is unable to return with any sense of pride to his job as a teacher in the Catholic school where this liaison had become known. Some things are not necessary for documentation, and if they are, they may not be necessary for dissemination.

Some participants in the treatment process not only have limited needs for information, they also need to have information limited. The busy primary care physician has little time in an era of increasing paperwork to review a 10-page single-spaced report on a patient, no matter how accurate or relevant. It is neither helpful nor effective to provide a general internist with a report which takes 15 minutes to review. It is far more likely that such a report will go unread, and that less information will be communicated, though at a very great cost, by such wordy communications. It may be necessary to gather information, but not to disseminate it. Dissemination of information must be done in a courteous way, attentive to the needs of the patient for privacy and the needs of the provider for relevant and sometimes only summary information.

The focus of treatment must be action. The managed care context is not suited to exploring rival diagnostic hypotheses and treatment considerations, nor in reviewing lengthy narratives that justify conclusions. The treatment team wants to know what to *do.* Defining a problem for a physician as follows is quick and meaningful: "The patient displays symptoms of a major depression likely requiring intervention with antidepressant medicines. Patient's sleep and energy pattern suggests a need for a more alerting medicine. Alcohol abuse seems a minimal risk, and the history of compliance is high. The recommendation is for a selective serotonin reuptake inhibitor." More information can be provided upon request or specific need.

Stating that "the patient appeared with symptoms of sleep and appetite disturbance following marital estrangement caused by a wife whose limited interest in her husband following the loss of children to maturity..." communicates little in terms of *what needs to be done.* The author of correspondence to physicians needs to recall that they are not defending a dissertation against critical eyes, but providing a conclusion to a colleague who respects their perception and who relies upon them to have done a competent diagnostic job.

DELIMITED TREATMENT

Managed care will be delimited care. Since managed care is conceived as a way of limiting the cost of services, it will certainly require various limitations. Several types of limitation, each likely to require some adjustment on the part of the therapist, will characterize managed care.

One delimiter will almost certainly be the amount of money spent to produce a treatment outcome, which will translate into some limitation in reimbursement for professional time. During the transitional time of managed care services, this likely will translate into brevity of treatment. Managed care programs in less sophisticated systems may merely limit the number of individual sessions authorized for a particular patient or a particular condition. More sophisticated managed care systems, such as closed-panel HMOs, may limit economic costs by providing programs that target specific populations with specialized interventions to achieve designated goals. At present, however, and probably for the foreseeable future, most outpatient care will be limited in duration.

The managed care therapist will need to be cognizant of limitations on time from the outset. Knowing that some degree of knowledge of the patient and rapport is necessary for efficient treatment, some time will have to be spent on gathering information and establishing a relationship. In so doing, the therapist can appraise not only what goals and which routes to achieve them seem most viable, but also which goals and forms of therapeutic relationships should *not* be pursued. Knowing and clearly defining the limitations on treatment with a client at the outset of therapy can help define the appropriate relationship between patient and therapist. In so doing, for example, a depressed patient with a very severe dependent personality disorder might more quickly be steered to less expensive groups or community support resources rather than encouraging a therapeutic dependency on an individual therapist to develop. Recognizing that depressions can occur in mild paranoid personalities, the managed care therapist might choose to play a more "consultative" role with such a patient, focusing on giving advice in a way that is more consonant with the patient's need for distance, cognitive rigidity, and wariness.

Not only are there limits in resources available to the patient, there are also limits in the nature of the relationship between the provider and the provider organization, on the one hand, and the patient, on the other. Psychology was once viewed as a "helping profession." Now it is considered as part of the "health care industry." With this change also come differences in the nature of the professional environment as well as in the relationships that can be offered to patients. Toennies (1940), the German sociologist, talked about the distinction between a "society" and a "community." The "community" can be illustrated by the values and relationships often attributed to the small town of years gone by. The system had a responsibility to the individual, and vice versa, which was rather global and general. In the "society," perhaps personified by the large anonymous city, the relationships between system and individual are more limited and specific, more contractual than caring.

While one can and should carry a spirit of community in relationships, the financial contracts between provider and patient will often be very limited and boundaried. This suggests that a patient may have many problems that are both unfortunate and potentially treatable, but outside of the scope of coverage and not of professional concern. The limitations in both reimbursement and relationships will likely cause tugs and tensions on the motivations of the professional and compassionate therapist.

7

Treatment for Major Depression

Major depressive disorder is defined by the diagnostic criteria of *DSM-IV.* It is a very prevalent and dangerous disorder. Although it may develop at any age, it usually begins in the mid-20s to mid-30s. While some people have only a single episode and return to their approximate level of previous functioning, more than half of those who suffer one major depressive episode will develop another. *DSM-IV* notes that of those who have two episodes, 70% will have a third, and of those who have three episodes, 90% will have a fourth. This means that the majority of those patients who have a major depressive disorder will qualify for the diagnosis of a recurrent major depressive disorder, either by history or by future course.

If episodes are untreated they often last for between 6 and 24 months, with the majority of patients returning to premorbid levels of functioning within two years (Goodwin and Jamison, 1990). Quick, spontaneous cures are not the rule. Weissman and Myers (1978) noted that in some of the epidemiological catchment area (ECA) studies, up to two thirds of the patients diagnosed with a major depressive disorder still had a mood disorder at one-year follow-up. Other studies have indicated that treatment for major depressive disorder is more effective earlier in the episode and that it may help prevent a chronic course (Kupfer, Frank, and Perel, 1989).

Major depressive disorder is seen in 2-3% of men and 4-9% of women at any point in time, with most estimates of overall prevalence at around 6% at any one time. Over the course of a lifetime between 7 and 12% of men and between 20 and 25% of women will experience major depression. There is some variability in diagnostic rates given the differences in populations studied, with some studies using those referred for treatment and others—like the ECA studies—relying upon screening data from the general population.

It is clear, however, that untreated major depressive disorder has a substantial effect on healthy functioning. Not only do family relationships suffer, but physical complaints are common and medical utilization increases. One study (Wells, Golding, and Burman, 1988) showed that 23% of patients with a major depressive disorder stayed in bed all or most of the day at least once in the previous two weeks, attributing this to their health, as compared to 5% of the general population. This same study showed that 48% of those with a major depressive disorder described their health as either fair or poor, as compared to only 19% of the general population. Broadhead, Blazer, George, and Tse (1990) reported that patients with a major depressive disorder experienced five times the disability days (11 as compared to 2.2) for a 90-day interval as the general population. Community surveys (Wells, Golding, and Burnam, 1988) also show that patients with a major depressive disorder display almost a 40% restriction in activity on an enduring basis.

Further, mortality rates secondary to suicide and accident rates are much higher with depressed patients (Wells, 1985). Patients with a major depressive disorder in the ECA study in one demographic group had a mortality rate that was almost four times higher than among nondepressed peer controls. Up to 15% of patients in the general population with major depressive disorders are psychotic. Some studies have even shown up to 25% of those patients who are receiving treatment for depression meet the criteria for a psychotic specifier (Spitzer, Endicott, and Robins, 1978).

The criteria for a diagnosis for a major depressive episode emphasize biological signs and symptoms, such as weight loss or gain, sleep problems, physical slowing, energy diminishment, and problems with concentration and thinking, as well as more mood-based symptoms such as anhedonia or depressed mood. It is with the major depressive disorders that many of the physical changes in brain functioning have been observed in advanced radiologic techniques, such as SPECT imaging. These studies of the brain (Schwartz et al.,

1994; Baxter et al., 1989; Baxter et al., 1990; George et al., 1995) show left prefrontal brain hyperactivity, blunted activity of events mediated through the limbic cortex, and differences in brain metabolism (Wu et al., 1992). Depression certainly appears to be a biologically involved condition, although, as noted, biological *causes* have not been demonstrated to the degree that biological *correlates* have been established.

USE OF MEDICATIONS

It has also been established, particularly for those with moderate to severe major depressive disorders, that medications are indicated as a treatment consideration. The Depression Guideline Panel (1993) contend that such severely impaired patients are appropriately treated with medication, whether or not formal psychotherapy is also used. They conclude that psychotherapy alone is not recommended for the acute treatment of patients with severe or psychotic major depressive disorders. This is based mainly on the lack of research validating the effectiveness of psychotherapy with such severe disorders and the proven effectiveness of medicines for groups of patients with these diagnoses. There does seem to be a standard of care which demands at least consideration of antidepressant medicines for severe, if not the less severe, major depressive disorders.

It is our view that different interventions have different ranges of applicability, and that biological interventions should be considered early on, in moderate to severe major depressions. As will be discussed, biological interventions do not preclude the use of other therapeutic efforts, and adherence to prescription medicine schedules may depend on patient monitoring in a therapeutic context. The use of medicines or other physiological interventions does seem to be a necessary, if not sufficient, aspect of treatment with many patients, however. It behooves even the nonmedical therapist to be somewhat knowledgeable about the medicines and other biological interventions used for treatment of depression. Although understanding will certainly increase with further research efforts and improved analytic techniques in radiological and biochemical investigations, some current themes in and the history of the use of medicines are worth discussion.

Long-term use of reserpine has been observed to cause symptoms of depression, attributed to the resulting depletion of certain neurotransmitters. Initially, the medicines categorized as monoamine oxidase inhibitors (MAO inhibitors) were thought to counteract this effect and they are still effective for the treatment of depression. Those who enjoy both serendipity and metaphor appreciate the fact that the MAO inhibitors were initially developed by the Germans for use as rocket fuel. Modified later for intervention with tuberculosus, they were found to also have an unanticipated effect on depression (Klerman, 1979). Use of these medicines led to the view that certain neurotransmitters seemed to be a component of depression, particularly norepinephrine (NE), serotonin (5HT), and dopamine (DA). While it remains unknown if increasing the somatic levels of these neurotransmitters is a primary mechanism for therapeutic intervention or only the first step in a complex reregulation of neurotransmitter systems, people did seem to get better on the MAOs.

The problem with the use of MAO inhibitors was not their effectiveness, but their side effects and the risk of toxicity. People who used the MAOs might often have gotten better, but they had to observe the complex restrictions, when using these medicines, that made compliance a problem. For example, certain tyramines, as found in some dairy products, red wine, and many other foods, are incompatible with this medicine. Treatment required patients to become aware of and adhere to dietary restrictions while simultaneously taking these medicines regularly.

New medicines were developed, the tricyclic antidepressants (TCAs). These, also, were effective in treatment of major depressive disorder for many people, and they are still in use, accounting for 50% of all antidepressant prescriptions written in the United States and Canada (Richelson, 1994). Many consider them to be more effective for severe depressions than the newer medicines, the selective serotonin reuptake inhibitors (SSRIs) (e.g., DeVane, 1994), but perhaps only because extensive research on the use of newer medicines with severe and psychotic depression has not yet been completed.

These tricyclic medicines also have side effects, among them cardiotoxicity. The risk of overdose is great, and it has been estimated that between 100 and 150 deaths per million prescriptions occur largely through such effects on the heart. These medicines also have a number of side effects that interfere with compliance, including anticholinergic effects, such as blurred vision, dry mouth, constipation, sexual dysfunction, and urinary retention; antiadrenergic effects, such as dizziness, certain forms of tachycardia, and effects on blood pressure; and antihistaminic effects, such as weight gain, sedation, and a lowering of blood pressure. TCAs can also interact with other drugs, for example potentiating the effects of certain antihypertensive medications. Patients taking these medicines are often less depressed, but complain about sedation, blurred vision, dry mouth, weight gain, sexual impotence, and other such symptoms which pose not only an inconvenience but also a safety risk for patients who depend upon alertness and agility.

New generation antidepressants began to appear in the 1980s, heralded by such medicines as Ludiomil (maprotiline) and Desyrel (trazodone). These produced both therapeutic benefits and better side-effect profiles, as well as major improvements in safety margins as a result of reduced toxicity and risk of overdose. These medicines also worked in slightly different chemical ways, blocking the reuptake of serotonin selectively, effecting certain 5HT 1A receptors. Though still sedating, these medicines tended to cause fewer anticholinergic symptoms, such as dryness of mouth. These medicines also started a research focus on serotonin and serotonin reuptake blockade in the late 1980s. Beginning in 1987 eight new medicines were introduced, including Prozac (fluoxetine), Zoloft (sertraline), and Paxil (paroxetine), called selective serotonin reuptake inhibitors, or SSRIs. New medicines now include Effexor (venlafaxine), Serzone (nefazodone), Wellbutrin (bupropion), with others to be released soon.

The newer medicines have been found to be effective in treatment of major depressive disorder, particularly in the less severe and nonpsychotic varieties (see, e.g., Osser, 1993; Dubovsky and Thomas, 1995). They also produce fewer side effects. Anticholinergic side effects are greatly diminished, as are sedation and orthostatic hypotension. The biggest benefit of these medicines, however, is best summarized by Joseph Talley (1994), who describes them as "idiot proof." They have less risk for overdose with far less cardiotoxicity. Once daily dosing increases compliance for Prozac, Paxil, and Zoloft, and dosages are fairly easy for the primary medical practitioner to calculate.

These medicines have truly become popular. Prozac is one of the most prescribed medicines in the United States, and the Facts and Comparisons newsletters report up to 33 uses of Prozac other than the FDA-approved indications for depression, obsessive-compulsive personality disorder, and bulimia. Prozac is being used for such conditions as premenstrual syndrome (PMS) and even experimentally with certain forms of arthritis and other physical conditions.

The new medicines are not without their drawbacks, however. The incidence of sexual side effects is a notable problem. Although initially sexual side effects were thought to be fairly rare and were so publicized by the drug manufacturers, some studies show between 20 and 70% of people taking these medicines have difficulty experiencing a sexual climax or maintaining much interest in sexual activity. This problem obviously affects compliance. Even some mild extrapyramidal side effects are noted, such as tremor and a sense of physical restlessness, called akathisia. In fact, when Prozac was originally blamed for some patient suicides, although this was disproven in subsequent studies, akathisia was thought to be a possible cause, since some patients have difficulty tolerating it. Other users experienced problems with insomnia, agitation, and an increase in anxiety or energy level. Some patients also reported an increase in gastrointestinal disturbance, and up to a third experience nausea when starting these medicines. Others experience headaches when taking these new antidepressants.

A newer medicine, Serzone, seems unique in affecting the 5HT-2 receptor site and having a demonstrated therapeutic benefit. Although requiring twice-daily administration, Serzone has a low incidence of sexual side effects, causes less nausea, and seems to reduce anxiety. It is hard to predict which medicines will evoke which side effects in any one individual, but some side effects often occur. Although side effects are reduced with the SSRIs compared with the older tricyclics, these new antidepressants are still no "magic pill."

Serotonergic agents may trigger what Lejoyeau, Ades, and

Rouillon (1994) have referred to as a "serotonin syndrome." The serotonin syndrome includes diarrhea, confusion, restlessness, hypomania, myoclonus, and sometimes lack of coordination and fever. Seizures, and even death, can result from this idiopathic and rare reaction, which is sometimes seen with combinations of antidepressants or following changes of antidepressants without an adequate "wash-out" from the previous prescription. Others suggest that medicines such as Seldane (terfenadine) and Hismanal (astemizole) may interact poorly with the SSRIs. Still, in spite of these rare complications or the even more common minor side effects, these medicines have been well tolerated by millions of patients with comparatively little in the way of physiological side effects.

Particular antidepressant medicines are chosen on the basis of side effects, since no antidepressant medicine has been shown to be clearly more effective than another, and no single medication results in remission of symptoms for all patients. Considerations of both short-and long-term side effects, previous positive response to a particular medicine, how first-degree relatives respond to a specific medicine, and medical status are involved in choosing a specific medicine. Antidepressant medicines used in psychiatric settings are significantly effective, ranging from 50 to 70% effectiveness for some populations, as compared with placebo rates of perhaps one out of three (see, e.g., Holister, 1994).

ELECTROCONVULSIVE THERAPY

Among the other biological interventions for treatment of depression, electroconvulsive therapy (ECT) has been proven effective in severely symptomatic patients who have failed to respond to one or more medication tryouts. It appears appropriate to consider ECT for patients with severe and/or psychotic depressions whose medical status indicates that it may be safer than medications or for those who have not responded to other forms of treatment. Particularly when hospitalization is indicated, as for the acutely suicidal or dangerously delusional patient, the use of ECT has been encouraged in managed care since it often resolves symptoms more rapidly than medication does. There are drawbacks to ECT, including the risks that occur with the use of any anesthetic, and the significant side effects include retrograde and anterograde amnesia. The research, however, finds ECT to be a very viable treatment alternative, far less malevolent than movies or folklore might suggest. Many patients improve significantly with few residual ill effects after this treatment.

The fatalities associated with ECT are rare. Kalinowsky (1975) found that more than 100,000 treatments with ECT resulted in a death rate of .003%, even though many of the patients in this population were elderly and had medical and cardiovascular problems that might place them more at risk. The use of muscle relaxants and anesthetics reduced the subjective distress and physical trauma associated with the older techniques, and modifications in techniques, such as unilateral rather than bilateral ECT treatments, may reduce memory disruptions (Zavodnick, 1990).

The majority of patients appear to respond to six to eight ECT treatments. Some find a high recurrence rate, perhaps as high as 50%, one to two years following ECT (Benbow, 1987). It should be recalled, however, that ECT is primarily used in acute treatment, and seems indicated more in severe, extremely severe, and psychotic forms of major depressive disorders. Most, yet not all, agree with Coppen et al. (1981) that the use of pharmacotherapy following the ECT substantially reduces the recurrence rate. As perhaps with other biological interventions, ECT is best utilized along with medicines or psychotherapy to enhance compliance and to help monitor recurrence. Although some (e.g., Grunhaus and Pande, 1994) argue for the possible use of maintenance ECT in those patients shown to respond favorably to it, most see it as indicated for the acute phase of treatment as only one component of an overall treatment plan.

The American Psychiatric Association developed a task force report in 1990 on the use of ECT (American Psychiatric Association, 1990) which confirmed the applicability of ECT to severely impaired populations, with both major depressive and bipolar disorders of mood. The uses of ECT, though limited, are well justified by the outcome literature. Grunhaus, Pande, and Haskett (1990) discuss the appropriateness of an ECT-specialty team and the use of specific protocols such as that developed at the University of Michigan for their ECT program. Perhaps applicable only to a small percentage of patients with very severe mood disorders, there is a place in managed care for electroconvulsive therapy.

LIGHT THERAPY

Light therapy is a well-documented treatment alternative for mild to moderate *seasonal* depressive episode. As noted in the diagnostic literature, a seasonal specifier can be added to a diagnosis of major depressive disorder. This usually occurs during the winter and is more commonly found in the northern latitudes with their long winter nights. The manifestations include a lack of energy in the winter, even when the patient sleeps more than in the summer; morning hypersomnia; weight gain in the winter, with a preference for carbohydrates; and weight loss in the spring, when fruits and vegetables are preferred and sleep returns to a normal cycle. A seasonal mood diagnosis can be made only if the symptoms are recurrent and the seasons are related to the onset of a major depressive disorder.

Melatonin, a neural transmitter produced in the pineal gland, has been implicated in seasonal depression. Melatonin is derived from serotonin, a neurotransmitter commonly the focus of studies on major depression. Exposure to sunlight suppresses the production of melatonin, which is made only during the night. Not everyone is affected in the same way by melatonin variation. Lewy (1994) estimates that 5% of the American population have a severe form of seasonal depression, with perhaps another 15% having a subsyndromal form. Before menopause, women seem to be four to five times more at risk for seasonal depression than men. After menopause the prevalence rates for men and women are more nearly equal. Light therapy seems indicated for those who have an authentic and well-documented case of a seasonally related recurrent major depressive disorder. Not any exposure to light will do. Exposure through the eyes at a 45-degree angle is indicated. Broad-spectrum light seems effective, yet certain wavelengths of white light have been found to produce greater suppression of melatonin than others. Light needs to be at a fairly high intensity, often up to 10,000 lux (ordinary room light is 200 lux, with bright artificial light about 2,000 lux). The intensity of 10,000 lux is comparable to the light of a cloudy day, as compared to a bright sunny day, which might produce a light intensity of 100,000 lux.

The use of light therapy necessitates some technical considerations and an awareness of possible side effects. The *DSM-IV* diagnostic criteria for a substance-induced mood disorder, for example, include the note that some somatic therapies used for depression, including light therapy, can induce manic-like mood disturbances. Light treatment has more than just a placebo effect (e.g., Brown, 1990), however, and, perhaps in conjunction with SSRI antidepressants, may be a very effective treatment (see Oren & Rosenthal, 1992; Campbell et al., 1995).

PSYCHOTHERAPY

Psychotherapy has a role in the treatment of major depressive disorder. Its effectiveness is substantiated in the research more for mild to moderate major depressive episodes than in the severe or psychotic depressive disorders. A number of studies have shown that psychotherapy alone is generally as effective as medicines in acute-phase treatment or with mild to moderate conditions (e.g., Beck, Hollon, Young, Bedrosian, and Budenz, 1985; Weissman, 1979). It has been suggested that psychotherapy in combination with medication may also help to enhance symptom relief by giving attention to secondary psychosocial problems or improving patient compliance (Rush, 1986).

BIPOLAR DEPRESSIONS

It should be recalled that depression can occur in a bipolar disorder, and a correct diagnosis is important. That a patient presents as depressed does not in and of itself indicate a history of recurrent depressions or of more manic episodes. Bipolar disorder refers to episodes of major depression interspersed with one or more episodes of mania or hypomania. There is disagreement about whether recurring depressive illness and bipolar disorders are distinct diseases. Frederick Goodwin, senior science advisor for the National Institutes of Mental Health, says that viewing them as totally separate diseases "simply doesn't stand up to the data," including the data on responsiveness to lithium carbonate (Goodwin, 1994). The "classic" bipolar disorder is now called a bipolar I disorder. The condition is generally thought to be equally prevalent between men and women, with the prevalence rate of .04 to 1.2%. This would indicate a "high end" estimated prevalence rate for bipolar disorder of approximately 1/10th of that for major depressive disorder.

Some writers disagree with this prevalence data. Goodwin (1994) estimates that depressive illness accounts for two thirds of severe major mood disorders, with bipolar disorder accounting for up to one third. He believes that bipolar disorders are underestimated because hypomania is often overlooked or undetected. He cites an NIMH study which showed that an appropriate diagnosis was not made in half of the patients with bipolar disorder, largely because of relying upon the patient for information. Goodwin notes that many patients remember hypomanic times as good or normal times, not as disordered times. An accurate diagnosis is important with such severe mood disorders, since some patients with bipolar disorder who are placed on tricyclic antidepressants may experience a manic response. In depressive mixed states antidepressants can cause agitation and increased insomnia and risk of suicide. Further, it appears that once antidepressants are used, later response to lithium is poor, suggesting that the inappropriate use of the tricyclics, and possibly of other antidepressants, induces resistance to lithium (see, for example, Wehr and Goodwin, 1987; Kupfer, Carpenter, and Frank, 1988).

The favorable response to lithium in early studies led to the popular clinical view that bipolar disorder has a good prognosis. This now seems not to be the case. Bipolar disorder is in fact a recurrent disorder. Some recent studies show that patients with bipolar disorder had significantly worse work functioning at follow-up than patients with unipolar disorder. One study found that two thirds of patients with bipolar disorder experienced deterioration of work status, and 45% were separated or divorced during the course of their illness. Women with bipolar disorder who do not receive adequate treatment live nine years less on average than expected and lose 12 years of normal health (Goldberg, Harrow, and Grossman, 1995; Solomon, Keitner, Miller, Shea, and Keller, 1995). It is estimated that 10 to 15% of untreated patients commit suicide, a rate 15 to 20 times the suicide rate of the general population (Depression Guideline Panel, 1993). Delusions and hallucinations are also common in the manic state.

Bipolar disorder appears to be less responsive to lithium than was formerly observed. Although the classic studies suggested either a partial or complete response in 80% of patients within the first year of use of lithium, more recent studies show a response rate of less than 50% today (Page, Benaim, and Lappin, 1987; Post, 1995). There are many possible causes for this apparent change. Goodwin (1994) notes that more than 50% of patients with a bipolar disorder have a history of drug or alcohol abuse that may affect the nature of their depressive episodes. Cocaine use may cause bipolarity in some mood disorders. The use of antidepressant medicines instead of mood stabilizers in misdiagnosed disorders may also contribute to the reduced effectiveness of lithium.

Robert Post (1994) discusses how poor compliance with lithium can cause refractoriness induced by discontinuation. Patients who initially respond well to the medicine and then stop taking it may no longer respond well when they resume the lithium. Post argues that if a psychotropic medicine is working, it should be only very cautiously discontinued, particularly in conditions with recurrent episodes, states such as bipolar disorder. Further, there is some thought that nonresponsiveness secondary to poor compliance may also occur with tricyclics. One article (Rapport and Calabrese, 1993) reports acquired tolerance to Prozac.

Taken together, these data suggest that both providers and patients are responsible for the reduced effectiveness of these medicines with mood disorders. Practitioners who assess bipolar disorders incompletely and prescribe antidepressants, patients who misuse drugs such as cocaine, poor compliance with prescibed regimes, and inadequate monitoring may well result in biochemical alterations in the neural chemistry of the brain which render mood stabilizers and perhaps antidepressants less effective than in the past. The authors find it interesting that there seem to be few, if any, reported cases of bipolar disorders with rapid cycling before the advent of tricyclic antidepressants and the rise of popularity of cocaine in our culture.

Fortunately, other medicines have been found to help in the treatment of bipolar disorders. Lithium is the initial intervention of choice, perhaps due to the wealth of early research justifying it. Certain seizure medicines are found particularly helpful in treatment of bipolar I disorders. Carbamazepine, with a trade name of Tegretol, seems to be as effective as lithium in acute mania, and perhaps involves lower relapse rates (e.g., Gerner, 1993). Some believe that compliance issues with adolescents justify carbamazepine as the mood stabilizer of choice with this population. Valproic acid, marketed as Depakote, also compares with lithium in treatment of acute mania (Freeman, 1992).

These medicines may cause a number of side effects. For example, verapamil, marketed as Calan or Isoptin, a calcium channel blocker used in the treatment of hypertension, has been found comparable in effect to lithium in some studies, but it poses some noteworthy though rare medical risks, such as congestive heart failure. Robert Gerner (1993) recommends that lithium be the first choice, except with geriatric patients, patients with any organic mental syndrome (who tolerate lithium poorly), or rapid cyclers. Seizure medicines may be tried next. ECT is also an option for treatment of bipolar disorders.

Medications work only when the patient takes them as prescribed. Compliance with prescription regimens, sometimes referred to as adherence to prescription schedules, is vital. The therapist in managed care may play a pivotal role in biological therapy by promoting compliance. Research indicates that compliance with treatment using medicines is quite poor, even worse than what patients report to their prescribing health care provider. One study showed that only 40% of general medical patients took more than 75% of prescribed medications, and almost 25% did not even get their prescriptions filled (Zoega, Barr, and Barsky, 1991). Another study found that more than half of a group of Southeast Asians had no detectable antidepressant levels in their blood despite self-reports of compliance (Kroll et.al., 1990).

The rate of compliance with medicines can be improved by effective and directed therapeutic efforts that acknowledge and attempt to resolve adherence difficulties. Verbal and written commitments by the patient to adhere to prescription regimens improve compliance (Putnam, Finney, Barkley, & Bonner, 1994). Reducing the complexity of prescription schedules, for example from three doses a day to one, may improve compliance (Conn, Taylor, and Kelley, 1991). Simpler instructions, communication styles that are sensitive to patient attitudes, rewards for patient compliance and reminders to take medicines increase compliance (Holloway, Rogers, & Gershenhorn, 1992; Spilker, 1992; Woody, 1990). Education about medicines is highly effective in enhancing compliance (Peet and Harvey, 1991; Youssel, 1983). Use of compliance- and adherence-enhancing strategies is effective, reducing noncompliance by more than 50% even in long-term patient populations (Lee, 1993). A continuing relationship with a patient which allows the therapist who monitors the medicine to explain side effects, reinforce and support conscientious use of medicines, inquire about problems, and encourage continuation is vital. The managed care therapist can certainly fill this role.

Poor compliance rates may explain the very poor outcome studies for use of antidepressant medicines in naturalistic, rather than more controlled, research studies. Brugha and Bebbington (1992) found that prescribing antidepressant medicines did not affect clinical outcome during a four-month follow-up period in a study of 115 patients. Physicians prescribing inadequate dosages or not monitoring compliance could have contributed to this phenomenon. "Real life" may be in sharp contract to the controlled and more closely monitored conditions of research studies on patient compliance with medicines. Monitoring compliance is a vital component to treatment with medicines, necessitating an interpersonal relationship which allows for monitoring, within the context of a structured program, to "manage" this therapeutic outcome.

This presents a challenge particularly with recurrent conditions, such as major depressive and bipolar disorders. A medication is prescribed for patients when they are ill which helps them feel better. When they are well, however, the side effects make them feel worse. This poses a long-term problem, especially since discontinuing medicines when they are working may cause them to be ineffective when they are needed again.

Compliance problems are more understandable when one considers some of the side effects of antidepressants. Examples can be found in Table 1. Few patients will experience all of the side effects with any particular medicine, but there are areas of significant risk and a likelihood of certain problems. Side effects have a direct influence on compliance. A study using patients for whom antidepressants were prescibed and using measures of blood serum antidepressant levels rather than patient report, found that 45% of those for whom certain medicines (amitriptyline and imipramine) were prescribed were noncompliant, while only one in twelve of those for whom a medicine with a more benign side-effect profile (desipramine) was prescribed were noncompliant (Boza et al., 1989).

Side effects, such as sexual dysfunction with the SSRIs, may seem inconsequential to patients who are depressed and uninterested in sex or almost any other interpersonal activity. As they become more active and involved in life and relationships, they might have a very different view toward sexual functioning. Going to the bathroom often or experiencing some tremor may seem a small price to pay for early release of a patient with mania from the hospital, but it can become a notable problem when that person returns to work in a sales position with long road trips and a visible tremor when he or she points to graphs and charts during sales meetings. Discussing these questions carefully and completely with patients before the fact may help them to realize that they are "signing on for the duration" and appreciate the implications of a commitment to take certain medicines, particularly the mood stabilizers.

While medicines are a treatment option for depressive and bipolar disorders, it should be remembered that the significant minority, perhaps later to become a majority, of patients do not respond well to medicines. This indicates that psychotherapeutic techniques need to be employed, perhaps in combination with medications. Since medications may not work with some patients, psychotherapy may be not only the preferred, but the *only* choice for intervention.

TABLE 1

Antidepressant Medicines and Common Side Effects

Drug	Anti-cholinergic	Central Nervous System		Cardiovascular		Other	
	dry mouth, blurred vision, urinary hesitancy, constipation	drowsi-ness	insomnia/ agitation	hypo-tension	cardiac arrhyth-mias	gastro-intes-tinal	weight gain
Amitriptyline (Elavil)	4+	4+	0	4+	3+	0	4+
Desipramine (Norpramin)	1+	1+	1+	2+	2+	0	1+
Doxepine (Sinequan)	3+	4+	0	2+	2+	0	3+
Imipramine (Tofranil)	3+	3+	1+	4+	3+	1+	3+
Nortriptyline (Pamelor)	1+	1+	0	2+	2+	0	1+
Protriptyline (Vivactil)	2+	1+	1+	2+	2+	0	0
Trimipramine (Surmontil)	1+	4+	0	2+	2+	0	3+
Amoxapine (Ascendin)	2+	2+	2+	2+	3+	0	1+
Maprotiline (Ludiomil)	2+	4+	0	0	1+	0	2+
Trazodone (Desyrel)	0	4+	0	1+	1+	1+	1+
Bupropion (Wellbutrin)	0	0	2+	0	1+	1+	0
Fluoxetine (Prozac)	0	0	2+	0	0	3+	0
Paroxetine (Paxil)	0	0	2+	0	0	3+	0
Sertraline (Zoloft)	0	0	2+	0	0	3+	0
Monoamine Oxidase Inhibitors	1	1+	2+	2+	0	1+	2+

0 = absent or rare   1+   2+ = in between   3+   4+ = relatively common

Adapted from Depression Guidelines, 1993

Psychotherapeutic interventions for mood disorders are presented in the next chapter, and questions of refractory disorders of mood are discussed subsequently. In spite of the hope that medicines can "fix the problem" with mood disorders, and the development of even more sophisticated antidepressants and more elegant mood stabilizers, there are inadequacies with a purely biochemical approach to mood disorders.

8

Treatment for Less Severe Mood Disorders

Dysthymic and cyclothymic disorders are the "minor league" variations of major depressive and bipolar disorder. They tend to be less severe, though more chronic. They might be considered the "dripping faucet" of mild chronic mood disorders, as compared to the "broken pipe" of severe or psychotic major mood disorders. Still, the social cost and personal difficulties associated with mild but more enduring problems may be more significant than for acute, more severe difficulties. Studies (e.g., Wells, Golding, and Burnam, 1988) reveal that more than a fourth of the patients with dysthymic disorder show a decrease in their level of activities. A significant percentage, almost one in six, report sometimes staying in bed the entire day, more than three times the rate of the general population. The diagnosis of dysthymic disorders in adults, for example, reflects behavioral patterns that have been present, without more than minor interruptions, for at least two years. This indicates a noteworthy and persistent degree of difficulty in functioning, perhaps accumulating over the years to greater "water loss" than might be experienced with the "broken pipe" problem of acute major depression. These mood disorders are "minor" only in terms of severity of symptom, not in terms of the consequences to patients or to the general population.

These more minor mood disorders were once regarded as behavioral, attitudinal, or even characterological. In fact, depressive personality disorder was proposed for further study but not adopted as a diagnosis in *DSM-IV.* This diagnosis would differ from dysthymic disorder in its emphasis on cognitive, interpersonal, or interpsychic personal traits. It was noted that "it remains controversial whether the distinction between depressive personality disorder and dysthymic disorder is useful" (*DSM-IV,* p. 732). The person with a depressive personality disorder displays low self-concept, a critical and blaming attitude toward the self, negative and judgmental attitudes toward others, pessimism, and excessive guilt.

The general view of the professional community is clearly that the minor mood disorders are caused more by psychological rather than physiological factors. The mainstream approach has accordingly been to use psychological interventions rather than the physical interventions used with the major mood disorders. This view is being challenged by empirical research, such as that conducted by David Dunner.(Dunner and Schmaling, 1994), which shows that dysthymic patients may respond well to selective serotonin reuptake inhibitors and that these medicines can be an effective component of their treatment.

Recent editions of the *DSM* have done much to enhance consensus and research by focusing on diagnosis based on symptom display rather than theoretical inference. For the practicing clinician, however, it may also be helpful to review dispositional response as a sort of "secondary diagnosis." For example, some patients with major depressive disorder do not respond to antidepressant medicines, indicating the need for other interventions, while some patients with dysthmic disorder may be responsive to antidepressant medicines. With further research the clinician might make the pragmatic diagnosis of a "medicine-responsive depression" versus a "medicine-nonresponsive depression" and design appropriate treatments based on likely outcome. Today this determination may be made on the basis of past treatment response, but future research may reveal which clusters of symptoms are more likely to respond to medicines than others. Until that time, interventions will probably be best selected on the basis of diagnostic categories articulated in *DSM-IV* and the patient's unique needs as assessed by the knowledgeable clinician.

In this chapter we describe a variety of approaches to specific symptoms, referring to interventions that might have a wide range of applicability. We are not proposing a "cookbook" of technical interventions. Rather, we are committed to a philosophy of respecting individual differences and the uniqueness of every person's social context and ecology. Diagnosis not only of a syndrome, but of the individual, is an inherent requirement of every one of these approaches. Although treatment should be "mechanical" in the sense that there are cause-and-effect relationships between therapist interventions and treatment outcomes, particularly in a managed care context, people are not machines. Accordingly, there is no single "tool" which will fix the problem of depression for everyone with a similar diagnosis. However, there is a wide range of tools that might be artfully used by the sensitive clinician to intervene in a task-focused way in order to help a specific patient with problems best categorized as depressive in nature.

We view treatment approaches with depression as falling into three broad categories: those that treat the syndrome of depression as an entity, those that treat specific symptoms constituting a mood syndrome, and those treatments that respond to factors seen as underlying causes for depression or mood problems.

The approaches that treat depression as an entity include those which rely upon the use of medicines, implying a physiological process which results in symptom clusters, and those that employ such approaches as psychoanalysis, which proposes that characterological or developmental problems create a pervasive dysfunction in the form of depression. The biological approach seems primarily useful with major depressive disorder, although perhaps it will also be found to be useful with certain forms of dysthymia, according to the work of Dunner noted earlier, among others. Dynamic therapies, even "brief" dynamic therapies, may tend to focus on the "depressive personality" or other reifications of symptom constellation. It is our view that the goal-directed and focused nature of the managed care treatment environment makes such a global psychotherapeutic approach less appropriate since vague treatment targets evoke general treatment strategies and very casually evaluated treatment outcomes. The managed care context will likely embrace specificity of goal in order to best manage limited resources. Accordingly, we will focus here upon interventions which address specific symptoms or underlying factors associated with mood problems.

A variety of symptoms constitute a syndrome in mood disorders. Low energy, appetite problems, sleep problems, feelings of hopelessness, and low self-esteem are among those noted for dysthymic disorder, while excessive goal-directed activity, restlessness, and other forms of sleep problems are components of cyclothymic disorder. Each of these specific symptoms can be targeted, and interventions can focus upon removing each symptom "one brick at a time" until the entire "wall" of the syndrome is gone.

LOW ENERGY

To address the problem with low energy an increase in physical activity may be effective. Physical exercise has been found to significantly reduce depression and anxiety (see Byrne and Byrne, 1993; Gleser and Mendelberg, 1990; Bosscher, 1993) and may even enhance the metabolism of antidepressant medicines (see, for example, de Zwann, 1992).

A study of depressed inpatients randomly assigned to short-term running therapy or "treatment as usual" were observed for eight weeks. The "treatment as usual" group did not display any therapeutic gains. Those doing the running improved significantly on measures of self-esteem, severity of somatic and psychological distress, body satisfaction, and general depression (Bosscher, 1993). Another study of college students aged 18–42 evaluated swimming as compared to weight training and no exercise controls. Both the aerobic and the nonaerobic exercise groups experienced a reduction in depression compared with the control group (Stein and Motta, 1992). Another study investigated hospital patients treated for major depressive disorder one to two years after discharge, assessing the usefulness of a regular aerobic exercise program. The subjects retrospectively ranked physical exercise as a most important element in their comprehensive treatment program. It is noteworthy that most continued regular exercise after discharge, and most of these exercised aerobically for at least two hours a week. Those who exercised tended to have lower depression scores in follow-up than the nonexercisers (Matinsen and Medhus, 1989). Lehofer,

Klebel, Gersdorf, and Zapotoczky (1992), reviewing psychological and biological research, discuss how running therapy can fit into psychiatric treatment for depression. An increase in activity level, improved social competency, and amelioration of a host of attitudes and habits associated with depression were noted as causes of improvement. An effect on vegetative symptoms of depression also stood out.

The Centers for Disease Control and the American College of Sports Medicine have formally recommended exercise for adults, specifically a total of at least 30 minutes of moderately intense physical activity every day, or at least on more days than not. The guidelines emphasize that exercise can be done in short bouts, for example walking upstairs instead of taking elevators. A variety of studies note that about 30% of adults have performed no leisure time physical activity in the last month. The new recommendations for adults in general recommend daily moderate exercise rather than vigorous regimented exercise but allow for intermittent exercise (Pate et al., 1995). Much of the research on exercise suggests that a treatment program for depression may require more sustained, aerobic activities.

Many patients who display low energy and other depressive symptoms are likely to be less inclined to exercise than a more energetic and goal-oriented person. The question is how to implement an exercise program for the depressed patient. Studies on adherence to such behavioral interventions provide some guidance. Dishman (1982) looks at adherence models of exercise that consider the exerciser, the exercise setting, and the interaction between the person and the setting as factors that affect recidivism in exercise programs. A review of such studies (e.g., Martin and Dubbert, 1982; Spevak, 1982) suggest that a buddy system and modeling are important, suggesting that a person is far more likely to start and to maintain an exercise program if he or she participates with at least one other person.

A social contract which encourages behavioral changes and a specific commitment agreed upon between patient and therapist can be important (see O'Brien, Petrie, and Raeburn, 1992). Involving family members in such activities as an evening walk, with a commitment not only with the patient but with the spouse or children, may be far more likely to result in compliance than merely advising a patient that exercise might be helpful. Following up on adherence tends to increase rate of compliance. Consistent monitoring of exercise regimens tends to reinforce the continuation of such programs. It has also been suggested (Martin and Dubbert, 1982) that personalized feedback is more effective than group feedback in adherence programs. Although exercise may ultimately become self-reinforcing for some patients, a great deal of extra energy on the part of the therapist may be necessary to "jump-start" this behavioral pattern.

SLEEP PROBLEMS

Sleep problems can be addressed in a variety of ways. Williams (1992) notes that "although some sleep disturbance associated with depression is undoubtedly biochemically based, sleep disturbance may, once initiated, be maintained by the maladaptive strategies the patient uses to try to cope." Behavior intervention may help the patient cope more adaptively by giving him or her more control over sleep onset. Lacks (1987) provides a good discussion of sleep physiology research and "sleep hygiene." She notes that there are many factors associated with sleeping disorders, including the sleep environment, the use of substances, sleep scheduling, presleep activities, daytime behaviors, and attitude toward sleep. Systematically dealing with each of these can provide a helpful approach to certain sleep problems. Lacks provides a summary of approaches, including attending to disruptions in the environment, such as the restlessness of a partner, the temperature of a room, or disruptive noises. A problem-solving approach is recommended. Attentiveness to caffeine consumption and other biochemical effects on sleep, including alcohol, can promote good sleep maintenance. Scheduling sleep in a consistent way such that circadian rhythm is not disrupted also can be beneficial. Presleep activities which help lower the level of arousal and reduce cognitive rumination may be helpful. Positive behavioral changes, such as increased exercise and general good health, can also help with sleep behavior. Borkovec and Boudewyns (1976) also recommend teaching relaxation exercises and greater stimulus control in a behavioral approach to sleep onset problems.

APPETITE PROBLEMS

Appetite problems somewhat resemble sleep problems in depression in that they may have a biological concomitant. Failure to attend to appetite and weight loss may help perpetuate depression. Patton (1993) discusses a variety of eating and appetite problems associated with depression: Physiological changes occur in response to food, affecting the level of appetite, the experience of hunger, or determination of satiation. Food may taste and smell different, and the patient may be less concerned about the effects of good nutrition or perhaps have other symptoms, such as anxiety, which affect appetite.

Patton also draws attention to the importance of excessive weight loss as a component to depression. Studies of starvation in prisoners of war and in eating disorders (Keys, 1950; Stunkard and Rush, 1974) show that a semistarvation diet can produce symptoms of depression such as irritability, depressed mood, loss of sexual drive, difficulties in concentration, and social withdrawal. Changes in food preference, such as the increased craving for carbohydrates noted in the seasonal mood disorder, discussed previously, point to a complex interrelationship between mood and eating. The research indicates that eating behaviors, if not appetite problems, can be monitored and addressed in a positive approach, which adds to the maintenance of overall wellness in the depressed patient. Certainly, there are special considerations and problems with the patient with an eating disorder who is also depressed which require specialized treatment. Many of the behavioral approaches to eating disorders may also be applicable to certain eating problems in the depressed patient. As the research indicates, specialized treatment of eating problems seems particularly indicated given the effects of eating behavior on mood disorders.

HOPELESSNESS AND LOW SELF-ESTEEM

Much of the theory about feelings of hopelessness and self-esteem in depression draws upon a common paradigm. Abramson, Metalsky, and Alloy (1993) posit a cognitive view of hopelessness that is quite similar to that proposed independently by Bernet, Ingram, and Johnson (1993) regarding low self-esteem. The former authors view hopelessness, and also low self-esteem, as stemming from an interaction between negative events and inferences about their causation. Abramson considers negative events an insufficient but perhaps necessary cause for hopelessness. In addition to having a negative experience, the depressed person either infers that the cause of the event is oneself, that the consequences are greater than they really are, or that the self is unworthy or deficient as a result of the negative event.

Bernet and colleagues (1993) refer to low self-esteem in a similar way. They regard the experience of a loss as a preliminary cause, with the attribution of the cause of the loss to oneself as a necessary secondary factor. Bernet discusses how self-esteem may be both cause and consequence of depression. Low self-esteem may predispose one to depression and may also stem from depression. Bernet also talks about vulnerability to depression, emphasizing cognitive factors, echoed by Abramson in some of his earlier work (e.g., Abramson, Alloy, and Metalsky, 1988).

Treatment for hopelessness and low self-esteem might challenge such thoughts about the negative events rather than focus on an unalterable past experience. Cognitive behavioral approaches which address the person's interpretation and thinking about a past negative event are likely to be more productive than focusing in an abreactive or cathartic way on the event itself. Challenging the patient's mistaken assessment of the consequences of a loss or pointing to other possible causes may be helpful.

Both of these viewpoints draw on the helplessness theory discussed previously. A lack of perceived control over the environment is clearly a factor in helplessness and low self-esteem. Interventions which alter a perception of the self as helpless may reduce the sense of hopelessness, improve self-esteem, and therefore alleviate depression.

Assertiveness training is frequently recommended as an aspect of the treatment for depression. Assertiveness reduces a self-perception of helplessness. This lends itself well to the managed care context, since there are some excellent self-help books on the subject, including *Your Perfect Right* (Alberti and Emmons, 1974) and *Don't Say Yes When You Want to Say No* (Fensterheim and Baer, 1975). Group approaches can also be quite effective in assertiveness training, teaching an individual to achieve better social outcomes by practicing better assertiveness in a group context. Feedback, encouragement, and an opportunity for rehearsal and monitoring are all aspects of group treatment. Specialized didactic classes in larger managed care programs can certainly be an adjunct in treatment programs not only for depression, but also for anxiety and certain marital problems.

Mastery experiences, which provide feedback to an individual on their capacity to exert control over their environment, can be quite helpful. As will be discussed in the chapter on children and adolescents, the Outward Bound training program is a good example of a program which helps individuals achieve real-life goals and overcome realistic physical challenges, thus changing their view of themselves.

Behavioral homework which brings about changes in one's environment may provide the feedback that it is possible for things to be different, producing an encouraging effect by its symbolic value in addition to the significance of the change itself. Interrupting habitual patterns of behavior, even in minor ways, can be quite effective in reminding the discouraged and depressed patient that change is possible. Bringing a few fresh flowers in a nice vase each week to a desk in a drab workplace, reorganizing the room of a child who has left home, or even cleaning and washing a car for the first time in months may constitute powerful statements made by the patient to him or herself that it is time to "get moving" and that movement is possible.

Of course, a focus on positive events, strengths, and past successes is incompatible with negative views of oneself as unalterably impotent or deficient. The research on depression suggests that encouragement may matter a great deal. Focusing upon the positive can be exceptionally helpful, both in treatment planning and in treatment strategy.

BEHAVIORAL APPROACHES

It is also possible to treat not merely the symptoms of depression, but some of the factors that may cause depression. This requires the use of theory as it can be applied to the individual's unique circumstances. Factors which serve as a foundation for depression may include cognitive mistakes or skill deficits.

Cognitive behavioral therapy is a structured approach to treatment of depression. Although a thorough discussion is beyond the scope of this book, there are a variety of excellent resources for the interested clinician (e.g., Beck, Rush, Shaw, and Emery, 1979; Meichenbaum, 1977). Cognitive behavior modification, as described in these approaches, attempts to alter specific mistaken habits of thought, ill-formed cognitive schemas, or mistaken inferences associated with depression. In this kind of therapy the therapist challenges assumptions and reviews events in the recent past which represent mistaken cognitive responses to unfortunate occurrences. Treatment is rather formal in some schools of cognitive behavioral therapy, but it is usually fairly short-term. Blackburn, Eunson, and Bishop (1986) examined only a 12-week treatment in one study, and considered patients nonresponsive if their depression was not profoundly improved in this time.

Williams (1992) discusses the importance of "socializing" the patient into a treatment approach. He recommends explaining to the patient that his or her own "negative propaganda" tends to discourage and demoralize. He provides some good examples of ways to make this approach more accessible and palatable to a patient who is likely to have had no previous experience of psychotherapy. Patient resources which emphasize the cognitive approach include David Burns' *Feeling Good: The New Mood Therapy* (1980) and Albert Ellis' *A New Guide to Rational Living* (Ellis and Harper, 1975). Such resources may be used to augment cognitively based therapeutic work.

Many of the behavioral approaches to treatment of depression are designed to increase the levels of activity and contingency-based reward in depressed patients. Perhaps the most notable is that of Peter Lewinsohn, discussed somewhat extensively in Chapter 3.

Lewinsohn's approaches have evolved over the years but initially included monitoring and increasing the rate of pleasant events. He has compiled a list of pleasurable activities which the patient ranks according to how enjoyable they were in the past, if they are enjoyable now, and how frequently they were experienced both previously and at present (Lewinsohn and Libet, 1972). Lewinsohn's approach attempts to increase the patient's frequency of engagement in activities that are likely to be intrinsically reinforcing or reinforced by others.

This approach can also be applied to enhancing patterns of self-reinforcement. If there are activities or events which are rewarding to an individual, these can be tied to other activities, such as work or other chores, creating contingency-based rewards, rewards which occur if and only if a behavior occurs. Scheduling a plan for reward and reinforcement with a patient, or perhaps with a variety of patients in a depression group, can result in an increase in pleasurable activities and in task completion, through the mechanisms of reward and reinforcement. Lewinsohn's excellent book, *Control Your Depression* (Lewinsohn, Muñoz, Youngren, and Zeiss, 1986), provides a host of resources for patients able to monitor activities and events, and explains the social learning model of depression.

Interpersonal approaches can certainly be helpful. Interpersonal therapy (ITP), discussed previously, is a focused and systematic approach to time-limited treatment which has proved helpful in the research on depression. Klerman, Weissman, Rounsaville, and Chevron (1984) provide a helpful perspective in their seminal book, *Interpersonal Psychotherapy of Depression*, which offers guidance and a formal approach to patient problems.

Marital and family therapy can be particularly powerful in the treatment of depression. Even behavioral approaches can allow partners to negotiate contracts so that each person can be more mutually rewarding to the other. Chronic problems with depression imply chronic problems with relationships, as well. Since it is difficult to segregate the emotional from the interpersonal, particularly in mood disorders, involving a spouse in treatment can be particularly helpful, both by enhancing the likelihood of change and by bringing the person's social context into focus in treatment. The evidence seems very clear that marital and family therapy can be especially useful with certain depressive problems and particularly, in our view, with chronic depressive problems.

Within the managed care context, it may be helpful to explain the need for systems-based interventions to administrators who view marital therapy as somewhat separate from individual treatment for depression. Listing such approaches as treatment for a patient's depression, with the spouse there for ancillary purposes, seems an honest and valid way to approach some complexities of reimbursement, more than justified by the research. It is hoped that the more sophisticated managed care programs will encompass the involvement of spouses and the use of marriage and family therapy in the treatment of chronic mood disorders. This approach may also prove beneficial to other members of a managed care population.

Increasing one's level and effectiveness in social functioning seems vital in the treatment of any recurrent depressive problem. It is well documented that the depressed patient has difficulties in social interaction, perhaps more pronounced the more intimate those relationships are. The loneliness of the depressed patient is often overlooked as a psychological construct, but it is important. In their excellent book, *Loneliness, Stress, and Well-Being: A Helper's Guide,* Murphy and Kupshik (1992) used a population of British subjects to show that social support and psychological well-being, as well as physical well-being, are connected. They propose ways to measure loneliness, providing a loneliness scale validated by research, and discuss how patients can be helped to overcome loneliness.

A component is the development of interpersonal skills. Objective skill deficits are better researched in American psychology than the phenomenological concept of loneliness, but these seem to overlap, and both appear to be quite relevant to depression. Helping patients become socially more adept and helping them to overcome loneliness may be much the same thing, and can help alleviate depression. Social competency often involves subtleties in human communication. Becoming attentive to social rules, norms, and folkways, including even such matters as physical distance in casual interaction, can be quite important.

Liberman, DeRisi, and Mueser (1989) describe ways to teach social skills to psychiatric patients. Although their book is more concerned with inpatients, it is applicable to outpatients, particularly those with personality and mood disorders. Their program emphasizes assessment and behavioral practice in a group context which allows feedback. They describe short- and long-term goals at both the instrumental and affiliative skill level. Affiliative, or social emotional, skills are those necessary to acquire and maintain deep friendships and family relationships. Instrumental skills are those used in social interactions which center around work and service relationships. Liberman and colleagues believe that skills targeted as goals should be "attainable, positive and constructive behaviors, specific, functional, consistent with the patient's rights and responsibilities, chosen by the patient, a high frequency behavior, and likely to occur in the near future." Their book is particularly recommended for those treating patients who may have chronic and severe social skills deficits.

Some may have deficits in social skills which are more acute and not characteristic of them prior to the onset of depressive problems. With those patients intervention may be easier. The authors are drawn to Adler's prescription for depressed patients (Adler, 1956), that they should do each day "three things to give another person pleasure." This is a wonderful example of ways to help a person become more socially reinforcing to others, and therefore more socially reinforced, as well as diverting the focus of attention away from the self to the external world. Focusing upon pleasure may help "open the door" to more spontaneous relationships rather than to perpetuate rigid and rule-governed behavior.

Monitoring expectations for goals and accomplishments seems to be an important component in the treatment of mood disorders. Self-perception is a cognitive act relevant to mood. A hypomanic patient seems excessively involved in goal-directed behavior while the depressed patient is less goal-directed than adaptive. The depressed patient has a diminished expectation for accomplishing tasks, and therefore seems to accomplish fewer of them, whereas the manic patient has a heightened view of one's capacity to accomplish tasks and tries to accomplish more of them. Expectations seem to be at the core of this, and these are a social as well as a psychological phenomenon.

Expectations develop when a person compares his or her performance against either a collective or an internalized standard for behavior. Negative self-evaluations may stem from a misperception of others or of self, or from a mistaken standard. Confronting an individual in a therapeutic way regarding his or her disparagement of self or others through unrealistic expectations may help to alleviate a depressive state. Often the depressed patient wants to be "gooder than good," and may become less depressed when encouraged to be "as good as most," yet allowed to be less than perfect.

BEREAVEMENT

Bereavement seems to require an exception to the focused approaches in managed care. A person experiencing and grieving a loss does best when ventilating emotions and expressing them to a confidant. While a therapist can certainly provide a safe environment for emotional expressiveness and healing, group therapy may provide an even more potent resource. Hospice groups, marriage transition groups, classes and discussion groups on empty-nest phenomena, and social groups for the recently widowed may provide both more meaningful and longer-term support than a managed care therapist who has been a stranger to the patient and whose involvement will end quickly. It may be that the managed care therapist is better able to help patients by referral and follow-up than by attempting to meet the patients themselves.

It should be recalled, however, that the emotional reaction of grieving may occur along with other life changes, since the person or the situation which has been lost to the bereaved patient may have been a functional as well as an emotional resource. Economic declines following divorce or retirement, a loss of social relationships as children age and parents become less involved in activities with other parents, and the loss of a specialized "work partner" due to the death of a spouse may constitute significant and difficult changes in life circumstances. It is important for the effective managed care therapist to attend to both the emotional and practical aspects of such transitions in an efficient and caring way.

9

Special Populations: Children and the Elderly

DEPRESSION IN CHILDREN

There has been much disagreement about the fact and the form of depression in children. Until fairly recently the majority opinion was that depression did not exist in children. Symptoms of unhappiness or demoralization were seen as reactions to life stress in a young child less able than an adult to weather the passing storms of situational despair. Psychoanalytic theories, in particular, proposed that depression could not occur in childhood. For example, Rie (1966) thought that the child's personality structure had not matured to the point where adult forms of depression could occur. Rochlin (1959) thought that depression could not occur until middle childhood because depression involved the superego directing aggression against the ego, a development not taking place until that point in life. Contrary views, such as Glaser's (1967), held that depression occurred in children but was "masked" and indirectly expressed. Glaser regarded such symptoms as somatic syndromes, phobias, and conduct problems as behavioral displays of underlying depressive problems. Early literature often suggested that depression could exist in children, but likely would not be directly expressed (e.g., Cytryn and McKnew, 1972).

Theory and research have evolved to the point that the majority of clinicians now believe that depression can exist in children. *DSM-IV* diagnostic criteria seem applicable, with few modifications, to children. *DSM-IV* notes that children and adolescents may sometimes have moods that are more irritable than depressed. Failure to make expected developmental weight gains may replace weight loss when not dieting as a criterion for depression in children. The diagnosis for dysthymic disorder shortens the criteria from two years to one, since chronicity has a different meaning for younger children than for adults.

The thinking has changed for a number of reasons. When the focus was on theory rather than signs and symptoms, it was hard to distinguish identical signs and symptoms that were observed in different underlying disorders. For example, conduct problems reflecting a depressive disorder were difficult to distinguish from conduct problems which resulted from a conduct disorder. It was also noted (e.g., Puig-Antich and Gittelman, 1982) that many of the symptoms that might be attributed to "masked depression" could potentially refer to all possible psychiatric disorders, making it hard to differentiate any condition from depression. With the development of a diagnostic nomenclature that relied more on descriptive than etiological issues, it was possible to refer to depression by reference to common symptoms.

Although different criteria for diagnosis other than those contained in the *DSM-IV*, such as Wing, Mann, Leff, and Nixon's (1978) Index of Definition, have been proposed, most find the *DSM* criteria best suited. These describe a cluster of symptoms sufficiently connected to constitute a syndrome of depression, equally applicable to children and adults. Puig-Antich, Blau, Marx, Greenhill, and Chambers (1978), using the Research Diagnostic Criteria (RDC) (Spitzer, Endicott, and Robins, 1978), a precursor to *DSM-III*, identified 13 children of elementary school age who met criteria for a major depressive disorder for at least a month. All were able to describe depressed mood and seemed to have a severe form of depression. Three had depressive hallucinations and 11 had suicidal thoughts. Carlson and Cantwell (1980) discovered that it may be common to see such syndromes in children who have been referred to psychiatrists, and Kashani, Holcomb, and Orvaschel (1986) have suggested that major depressive disorders can even occur in preschoolers.

Using these adult diagnostic criteria with children can be a challenge, however. Children may differ from adults in their ability both to experience and to report some symptoms. Cognitive features are an example. For a child to experience a sense of shame or guilt implies some development in cognitive ability, and relying on use of the concepts of failure and shame may necessitate that a child be well into school age (e.g., Harter, 1983; Rutter, 1986). Children may have difficulty reporting criteria accurately. They may have trouble differentiating basic emotions or may mislabel them, as noted by Kovacs (1986). Concepts of quantity and duration may also be harder for children to describe, making such things as recurrent depression hard to assess.

Some have proposed that the diagnostic criteria for depressive disorders be modified somewhat to take into account a child's level of functioning in the various cognitive and affective dimensions. Carlson and Garber (1986) proposed a way to assess differing base rates at different developmental stages. Their multitiered approach takes into account the varying prevalence of symptoms in children. Some indicators, such as suicidal thoughts, are found rarely in children. Others are more common in children, such as social withdrawal. Still others seem fairly unrelated to age.

Until such changes occur, the current nomenclature seems workable. Some, such as Ryan and colleagues (1987), have studied clinical populations of almost 100 children and adolescents with major depression. Measuring sign and symptom frequency and severity, they found no difference between children and adolescents in terms of overall severity of depressive symptoms. They did discover that prepubertal children had more somatic complaints, psychomotor agitations, phobias, hallucinations, and separation anxiety. Adolescents, however, had a greater sense of hopelessness and helplessness, experienced diminished capacity for pleasure, slept more, and used more alcohol and drugs. Carlson and Kashani (1988) compared a small sample of preschool children with a large sample of adults who had also been diagnosed with major depressive disorder. They discovered that adults were more likely to have anhedonia, diurnal variations, psychomotor slowing, hopelessness, and delusions. The children were more likely to have depressed appearance, low self-esteem, and somatic complaints. This has been questioned, however, by Mitchell, McCauley, Burke, and Moss (1988) and Kovacs and Paulauskas (1984), who found few differences in the symptoms of depression across different age groups. It should also be recalled, however, that a diagnosis of major depressive disorder requires some similarity of signs and symptoms among the subjects, so there would be limited differences in symptom display among the study participants. Still, research supports the application of the diagnostic criteria in the *DSM* to a variety of age groups.

The same holds true for bipolar disorders. Carlson (1990) has reviewed the literature on bipolar disorders in children. It is agreed that bipolar disorders can also exist in children, although symptoms change as children age. Older children, 9–12 years of age, seem to display more of the cognitive symptoms of a bipolar disorder, such as grandiosity, whereas younger children seem to exhibit more of the energetic physical display of hypomania, such as irritability and emotional intensity. Lewinsohn, Hops, Roberts, Seeley, and Andrews (1993) found a lifetime prevalence rate for bipolar disorder in adolescents similar to that of adults.

Some see it as a challenge to differentiate between hypomania and hyperactivity, as might be found in an attention-deficit/hyperactivity disorder (ADHD). Strober, Hanna, and McCracken (1989) noted that children with bipolar disorders tended to have more shifts in mood, may have experienced hallucinations or delusions, and were apt to be more goal-directed than hyperactive children. Coll and Bland (1979) agree that both mania and cyclothymia can occur in children, but saw more of a difficulty differentiating this from ADHD than did Strober, Hanna, and McCracken (1989).

Given the difficulties in diagnosis and some disagreement about what criteria to employ, it is not surprising that prevalence rates for depression with children should be as varied as they are. The prevalence rate has been estimated as 0.89% in preschool children, 2% in school-aged prepuberty children, and 4.5% in adolescents (Weller and Weller, 1990). Anderson, Williams, McGee, and Silva (1987) believe that 1 to 2% of children will experience a major depressive disorder by their teen years. Of interest is that boys and girls seem equally at risk for a major depressive disorder until puberty, after which girls become more likely to experience depression and maintain an increased risk ratio throughout their lives. Other studies show differing prevalence rates in different cultures, ranging from

1.7% in New Zealand to only 3 out of more than 2,000 in the Isle of Wight study (Rutter, Tizard, and Whitmore, 1970).

The difficulty of diagnosing children is more pronounced at younger ages than in adolescence. Increased attention to adolescent depression and suicide risk has prompted closer scrutiny of this age group. Peter Lewinsohn et al. (1993) studied a large population of rural and urban high school students, numbering over 1,700 at the entry of the study, with 1,500 still available for one-year follow-up. They found a very high rate of prevalence and recurrence of major depressive disorder in adolescents. In fact, Lewinsohn found a lifetime prevalence rate for depression of 27% in girls and 13% in boys, with less than a 1% incidence rate of bipolar depressive disorders.

A number of writers have commented upon the possible changing prevalence rate of depression over recent years (e.g., Schwab, 1993; Cantwell, 1994). Cohort studies show that rates of depression seem to be increasing. There are higher rates of depression in those born between 1950 and 1960 than in the 10 years before. Rates were higher still between 1960 and 1970. In fact, the mean age of onset of depression has dropped from approximately 40 years of age to the late 20s. It is frequently found in epidemiological studies that a shift in the age base towards younger age groups for any chronic or recurring disorder indicates future increases in the prevalence of the disorder. While many factors can account for this, such as greater acknowledgment of depressive symptoms and less stigma attached to emotional conditions, it still seems that there are causative factors for depression yet to be discovered. Given the rate of increase, faster than would be found in a condition responsive only to genetic increases, some psychosocial or environmental changes must be taking place.

The culture has changed. Divorce and family instability have increased during the last few decades, as has drug use among teens. Other biological mechanisms may be operating, such as the steady decline in the average age of menarche over the past century (Rubin, 1990). Whatever the factors may be, the risk for depression has increased over the last several decades. Although some of the research can be challenged on methodological grounds, some measures of depression have undeniably increased. For example, Shaffer

(1988) estimated that the rate for suicide risk among white males age 15–19 has almost doubled, a trend which is observable in several countries. Most of the industrialized world seems to be experiencing an increase in the rates of depressive disorders and an earlier age of onset, meaning that these conditions may significantly affect children and adolescents.

Understanding the significance of changing prevalence is confused by disagreements about diagnostic criteria, difficulties in assessment, and the challenge of differentiating developmental delays from depressive disorders. Adding to the complexity is the issue of comorbidity. Almost anyone who has written extensively about child and adolescent depression has acknowledged the very high rate of comorbidity between depression and other conditions, particularly alcohol and substance abuse. Fleming, Offord, and Boyle (1989) reported that more than 90% of those subjects with clear cases of depression also had a conduct or emotional disorder, or displayed hyperactivity or somatic symptoms. Rohde, Lewinsohn, and Seeley (1991) found 42% of adolescents with some form of comorbidity.

Diagnosis and treatment of depression need to take this comorbidity into account. Greenbaum, Prange, Friedman, and Silver (1991) studied a large sample of more than 500 adolescents aged 12–18 identified as having severe emotional disturbances. Depressive disorders were found to be among the disorders most strongly associated with substance abuse. Almost one half of those with severe depression also had substance-abuse problems. Milin, Halikas, Meller, and Morse (1991) found that 18% of adolescents who had abused either drugs or alcohol met *DSM* criteria for some form of a depressive disorder, compared with 5% of those who had not used drugs.

There was comorbidity with other conditions, as well. Ryan and colleagues (1987) found that moderate to severe separation anxiety was comorbid with depression in a majority of children and more than a third of adolescents. Strauss, Last, Hersen, and Kuzdin (1988) found that nearly 30% of patients with anxiety disorder had major depressive disorders. In a study of school refusers, Bernstein (1991) found that around half were depressed. Studies suggest that between 25 and 80% of eating disorders have concomitant depressive disorders (Strober and Katz, 1987). These findings are similar to those in adults with eating disorders.

It is not surprising that there are divergences among comorbidity estimates given the vast differences among the estimates of prevalence for depressive disorders. It can be surmised, however, that if a child or an adolescent is depressed, he or she is likely to have other problems as well. Children with depression are more at risk for alcohol abuse, particularly as they approach the teen years. They are likely to have behavioral problems, such as substance abuse, eating disorders, or conduct problems, and they are very likely to have a condition that will become chronic. In fact, there is even some suggestion that there is a higher rate of switching from depressive to bipolar disorders in childhood-onset depression than in adult-onset disease, projected as high as 37% in the Kovacs and Paulauskas (1984) study.

Although mood disorders may be somewhat hard to assess with children, they are worth assessing. Untreated childhood depression is likely to coexist with depression in other family members or will affect them. In a review of existing literature, McCauley and Myers (1992) found that depressed children were likely to continue being depressed into adulthood if untreated. Depression can reduce psychosocial effectiveness at an early age and is likely to become more recurrent and entrenched and to lead to other conditions, such as substance abuse or bipolar disorders, which have very poor prognostic outcomes and affect a child in the social, vocational, and health dimensions.

Assessment of Deprssion in Children

Assessment of childhood and adolescent depression requires particular tools and approaches. There are a number of interview and self-report measures for children and adolescents. The interview measures include the Child Assessment Schedule (CAS) (Hodges, Kline, Stern, Cytryn, and McKnew, 1982), a structured psychological interview designed for children between the ages of 7 and 12 years old. Modeled after *DSM-III*, the structured questions of the CAS focus on diagnostic criteria for a variety of childhood disorders, including depression. The interview consists of two parts. The first requires an individual to respond "yes" or "no" to an extensive number of questions. In the second part, the clinician separately records observations about the interview. Studies show fairly good interrater reliability and discrimination among various studied groups.

The Interview Schedule for Children (ISE) (Kovacs, 1981) is another structured interview which focuses on a wide range of *DSM* diagnoses, developed during the *DSM-III* era. The ISC focuses on current major symptoms of psychopathology and their severity, allowing for appraisal of mental status, behavioral observations, and clinical impressions. It also focuses on the phenomenology of various childhood disorders.

The Childhood Depression Inventory (CDI), modeled after the Beck Depression Inventory, is probably the most widely used self-report measure of depression in children (Kovacs, 1992). This instrument has been challenged in its diagnostic utility (e.g., Hodges, 1990), largely for its failure to assess the onset and duration of depression and for the inclusion of conduct-related items initially thought to reflect masked depression. Factors of acting out, dysphoric mood, loss of personal and social interest, self-deprecation, and vegetative symptoms have emerged from factor analytic studies (Craighead, Curry, and Ilardi, 1995). A recent study (Craighead et al., 1995) shows that the CDI total score may be a very practical measure for classifying children as depressed or nondepressed.

Many who work with children find it helpful to refer to the data from parents and teachers in making an assessment of overall functioning in developing a clinical diagnosis. We also recommend such an approach, but are well aware of the limitations of this in assessing depression. Clinical assessment often begins with parental interviews and proceeds to assessment of the child. There is some agreement that children do not provide as reliable information as do adults, particularly when it comes to their ability to focus on the signs and symptoms of depression. Children may not be able to make sense of the term "slowed down thoughts," perhaps not having a sense of the normal pace of cognitive functions.

There have been a number of studies on the agreement between parent and child reports of depressive symptoms (e.g., Barrett et al., 1991). These show a fairly low level of agreement. The Barrett study reported that the range of overall agreement on depressive symptoms, with both the child and adult agreeing on their absence or presence, range from 40 to 86%, with the majority falling between 60 to 70%. As Harrington (1993) points out, "Since one could achieve 50% overall agreement simply by tossing a coin, these results are not especially encouraging." Edelbroc, Costello, Dulcan, Conover, and Kalas (1986), examining the relationship between age of the child and level of agreement, found that there was better agreement between the perceptions of parents and older children than between the perceptions of parents and younger children.

Moretti, Fine, Haley, and Marriage (1985) found that parents' rating of their own depression correlated with the ratings of children's depression. McGee, Williams, Kashani, and Silva (1983) found a similarly strong relationship between a mother's level of depression and reports of a child's behavioral problems. Of note is that the mother's reports of behavioral problems were not confirmed by the child or the teacher, suggesting that parental reports may sometimes be more of a projection of difficulties due to some filtering of data on the part of the parent.

It seems wise to combine information from both outside reporters, such as parents and teachers, and from interview and rating scale information from the child in making the diagnosis of depression. Some symptoms, such as psychomotor retardation, may be better assessed by the outside observer. Below the age of 10 a child may have difficulty with the complexity involved in understanding some symptoms, meaning that more reliance should be placed upon adult reporters. Teachers, particularly experienced teachers, can provide good measures of behavioral observation.

Standardized measures, such as the Achenbach and Edelbrock (1983) rating scales, assess specific behavioral signs. Although not designed for depression, these scales can provide a quick measure of overall psychosocial functioning and open the door for the teacher or parent to provide additional information by letter or notation. A measurement of the child's overall level of psychosocial functioning is important, particularly in assessing the severity of any psychological condition. Standardized scales can provide some normative data to supplement the more specific symptom report made by the patient and parents.

Psychological treatments are generally favored over biological interventions with children and adolescents. In fact, controlled studies on the use of medicines for childhood depression have been unable to show any benefits beyond those that can be ascribed to placebo affect (e.g., Geller, Cooper, McCombs, Graham, and Wells, 1989; Puig-Antich et al., 1987). Treatment with electroconvulsive therapy with children has been found in at least one study (Carr, Dorrington, Schader, and Wale, 1983) to produce subsequent neuropsychological deficits, such as in auditory processing. There have been no long-term follow-up studies, however, to determine whether such deficits produced by ECT maintain or increase in months and years following administration of the therapy.

There have been studies to suggest that treatment with lithium and the anticonvulsants used as mood stabilizers may be helpful in treatment of severe bipolar disorder with adolescents, but there have been no systematic long-term placebo-controlled studies of lithium maintenance therapy. Some studies (e.g., Strober, Morrell, Lampert, and Burroughs, 1990) of the naturalistic data reveal a lower risk of relapse in patients with bipolar disorders treated consistently with lithium than in those who are clearly noncompliant, but the implications are far from clear. It is of interest that children with bipolar disorder in the Lewinsohn study were found to have more problematical behavioral patterns and to be at a greater risk of suicide than either matched controls or those with major depressive disorder. The current research justifies the use of lithium and other mood stabilizers with well-documented and severe cases of childhood and adolescent bipolar disorder, but not with other mood disorders in these age groups.

Given the high risk for depression in other members of the families of depressed children, it makes sense to consider family therapy in treating childhood depression. Family interventions can also help establish appropriate reinforcement schedules for prosocial and socially contributory behavior on the part of the parents. Family members control primary reinforcements for younger children and can encourage cooperative functioning at an early age. Even with adolescents, family intervention, or at a minimum, intervention involving parents, seems quite indicated with mood disorders and perhaps with other conditions. The theoretical and research support for early intervention with mood disorders certainly seem applicable to children, and a well-designed treatment program might allow intervention which also helps adult family members. Using the Adlerian model of family therapy, Croake (1987) has even shown that involving fathers who were hospitalized for depression in parenting training directed at mothers, reduced fathers' hospital length of stay and readmission.

Psychological therapies include a range of alternatives. For those situations where family therapy seems counterindicated or is not possible, cognitive or behavioral approaches may be appropriate. The Lewinsohn programs for behavioral control of depression have been found particularly helpful with children (e.g., Lewinsohn, Clarke, Hops, and Andrews, 1990). The programs include assertiveness training, increasing level of activity, and reward management. Their Coping with Depression Course for adolescents (Lewinsohn, Antonuccio, Steinmetz, and Teri, 1984) was found to be very effective in initial trials.

Cognitive behavioral therapy has been effective with young people, as found in a number of studies (Reynolds and Stark, 1987; Matson, 1989). Stark (1990) even uses techniques from Beck's Cognitive Behavioral Program to help a child to understand upsetting events better, to look at ways of altering automatic thinking patterns, and to learn that outcomes may be different than imagined. Of course, these techniques take into account the child's capacity for intellectual and interpersonal development.

Self-control and self-monitoring methods have been used with young children (Reynolds and Coats, 1986). Education in self-monitoring may include teaching a child to tell the difference between subtleties of emotions and enriching their "emotional vocabulary" (Stark, 1990). Self-evaluation training has been used with children who may have an idealized and unrealistic expectation for performance. If evaluating one's performance is done by comparing oneself to some standard for behavior, a negative evaluation can come from comparing adequate behavior to an inflated standard. Such negative self-evaluations are common symptoms of depression in children (e.g., Kendall, Stark, and Adams, 1990) and can be modified through deliberate treatment.

Moreau, Mufson, Weissman, and Klerman (1991) report several

cases of children and adolescents who responded to interpersonal therapy. Interpersonal psychotherapy seems particularly appropriate with depressed adolescents who are more involved with peers than younger children might be. Fine, Forth, Gilbert, and Haley (1991) use social skills training with depressed young people. Matson (1989) has given examples of case studies to show how social skills training can be quite helpful in specific cases of childhood depression.

Williamson, Birmaher, Anderson, Al-Shabbout, and Ryan (1995) found that stressful life events play a very important role in the development of depression in adolescents. They conducted a study in which they categorized stressful life events as "dependent" and "independent." The dependent life events were those over which an adolescent believed he or she had some control, such as a parent–child conflict. Independent life events were those that occurred without any influence of the adolescent, such as the death of a grandparent. Major depressive disorder was found to be associated more with dependent, rather than independent, events. Skills training to reduce the frequency or magnitude of stressful interpersonal conflicts seems warranted by this line of research.

Therapeutic outcomes can occur as a result of many therapeutic experiences, of which psychotherapy is only one. Life events can also have a beneficial effect. A number of programs provide significant psychological benefits for children and adolescents through various powerful life experiences. For example, the Beech Hill Hospital makes use of the Outward Bound Wilderness Survival Course as part of their substance-abuse treatment program. One study (Kennedy, 1993) shows that 91 adolescents, the majority of them males, who had been admitted to an inpatient treatment program, benefitted significantly from a wilderness survival program. One year after participating in the Outward Bound program, 47% reported complete abstinence from alcohol and other drugs. Further analysis indicated that the involvement in other adjunctive programs, such as the self-help programs offered by Alcoholics Anonymous, as well as severity of psychopathology and extent of prior drug use, also affected relapse rate.

Whether psychological benefits ensue from overcoming physical challenges in a team context or from the combination of such benefits with physical exercise is unknown, but both can be prescribed as behavioral interventions. MacMahon (1990) comments on the benefits of athletic participation, of less intensive forms of recreational play, or of less physically challenging programs than Outward Bound. Kiewa (1994) attempted to develop a theory of adventure experience in what was called "wilderness therapy." The powerful learning situation provided by the outdoors, as in the Outward Bound and similar programs, appears to enhance the participant's sense of self-control. Cooperation, an experiential learning base, intensity of feeling, success, choice, and an emotionally supportive climate have all been regarded as responsible for the demonstrated benefits of some of these programs. Although some question the long-term effects of these programs (e.g., Castellano and Soderstrom, 1992), combining such interventions with other forms of treatment and follow-up in a multimodal treatment plan can be powerfully effective.

A wide variety of life events can also help to challenge an adolescent's worldview, enhance his or her sense of competency, or enhance relationships with peers and other family members. Organized sports, church youth groups, and scouting may be beneficial to all children in a variety of ways. These activities may provide greater likelihood of social success in a structured and encouraging environment. Such opportunities may increase the level of a child's social activity, helping him or her to develop a more balanced approach to life and social relationships or a wider behavioral repertoire. Such programs may be very therapeutic, but therapy can be achieved far away from the therapy hour. Particularly in the managed care treatment context, the use of such ancillary resources seems indicated.

Summary

There has been very little controlled research on the various treatment modalities used with children. This is understandable given the complexities of children's natures and needs, the complications of diagnosis, and the varying kinds of depression in children and adolescents. Some conclusions seem clear, however. First, depression seems to exist in children. Second, *DSM* criteria seem appropriate in assessing it. Third, assessment can employ a variety of measures, including interview, parent and teacher surveys, questionnaires, and objective testing. Finally, with the possible exception of severe and well-documented bipolar disorder, depressive disorders in children do not appear to respond to medication. Psychological therapies do seem effective, and family therapy and counseling can be exceptionally helpful with childhood disorders of mood. Participation in positive life-changing events, such as wilderness programs, may be particularly effective in the brief treatment of depression under managed care.

DEPRESSION IN THE ELDERLY

The role of depression in the elderly, as with children, is often misunderstood. Raskind (1993) notes that a problem complicating diagnosis in the depressed elderly patient is the tendency to attribute signs and symptoms of depression to "just growing old." He observes that this mistake is commonly made by depressed elderly patients, family members, and even their physicians. One can think that as friends become infirm, spouses die, children move away, and the rewards and structure of work evaporate with retirement, that unhappiness, and even depression, are a predictable consequence. In fact, Palmore and Kiveh (1977), following a longitudinal study of elderly patients, concluded that satisfaction with life is not associated with aging itself. Epidemiological studies suggest that the prevalence of major depressive disorder in the elderly is less than 3%, with perhaps other mood disorders affecting 15% of the population, rates comparable to those of younger populations (Blazer, Hughes, and George, 1987).

Diagnosis of Depression in the Elderly

It is often hard to diagnose depression in the elderly, possibly because of some differences in the symptoms in this population. Elderly patients deny depressive signs and symptoms more often than younger patients (DeAlarcon, 1964), and they often present with physical concerns and signs. There are indications that depression is more likely to produce somatic symptoms in the aging. In one study (DeAlarcon, 1964), two thirds of elderly depressed patients had physical complaints as a presenting symptom. One study of a Veteran's Affairs Medical Center found that 20% of those receiving outpatient medical treatment met the criteria for major depressive disorder (Kukull et al., 1986). Although the *DSM-IV* criteria apply to the elderly, the physical signs of depression, such as physical slowing, fatigue, and weight loss, along with anhedonia, are more often observed than are mood problems. Those elderly patients focusing on somatic symptoms are often likely to deny or under-report sadness or disturbance of mood.

Williamson and Schulz (1992) show a relationship between medical symptoms and depression for the elderly. The total number of physical symptoms, as rated by the physician, was found to be the best predictor of depression, followed by the patient's report on the number of pain medications being used, the subjective evaluation of health, and restrictions on activity. Self-reports of health-related concerns, worries, and lack of social support also correlated with depression. Since hypochondriacal concerns are a significant predictor of suicidal risk in the elderly, it makes sense to draw less of a distinction between somatoform disorders and depressive problems in aging populations.

Depression is also a significant risk factor for mortality in the elderly. The mortality rate for depressed nursing home residents is twice that of nondepressed cohorts (Rovner et al., 1991). The risk of successful suicide is higher for elderly men over age 60 than for any other demographic group (Blazer, Bachar, and Manton, 1986).

Depression in the elderly is also poorly treated. In a study of nursing home elderly, Heston and colleagues (1992) found that even when depression is recognized by physicians and staff, treatment seems inadequate by most acceptable standards. Diagnosis is complicated by the fact that numerous medicines and medical conditions can produce depressive symptoms. Cardiological, pulmonary, and renal difficulties can cause sleep problems, diminished energy and vitality, or difficulties in concentration and attention. Medicines may help to treat these medical conditions, but they can also have effects resembling signs and symptoms of depression.

Depression is often mistaken for dementia in the elderly. Typical signs of depression, such as difficulty concentrating or a lack of interest and desire, get reported as poor memory, decreased ability to learn, and general forgetfulness. The medications used to treat a particular disease are sometimes supplemented by others, for treatment of their depressive side effects. The combination and number of medicines may also cause signs and symptoms of dementia.

Some research indicates that a diagnosis of dementia does not preclude a diagnosis of depressive disorder (Orrel and Bebbington, 1995). With dementia, factors of age, social class, severity of dementia, relationship with a caretaker, and changes in routine were associated with depression. It may be, in fact, that cognitive impairment and the diminishment of resources to ward off depression make depression more likely. Combined with the increased cognitive limitations and the dwindling of social support, dementia makes patients even more vulnerable to depression.

The first onset of a primary major depressive disorder after age 50 is fairly uncommon, and the Depression Guideline Panel notes that it is often related to a specific medical condition and thus requires careful medical evaluation (Depression Guideline Panel, 1993). Other elderly patients with depression are likely to have recurrent episodes, and some have bipolar disorders.

Treatment of Deprssion in the Elderly

Tricyclic antidepressants (TCAs) have been commonly used with the elderly to good effect. Veith and colleagues (1982) showed that the use of TCAs by depressed patients after heart attack or heart bypass surgery helped with the depression. However, Giardina et al. (1979) draw attention to the cardiovascular risks with TCAs. Orthostatic hypotension—low blood pressure—that can lead to balance problems and falls, is a relevant side effect of TCAs.

Those patients who take TCAs have been found to be 100% more at risk for hip fracture than those who do not (Glassman, Bigger, Giardina, and Roose, 1979; Veith et al., 1982). Boyer (1994) discusses the increased risk—estimated between 200 and 500%—for auto accidents with elderly patients taking antidepressants, pointing out that this issue may be relevant in claims of malpractice. Further, TCAs can impair psychomotor functioning and produce subtle cognitive problems in the elderly (Tiller, 1990).

Sometimes, however, these medicines are necessary, and if they are, nortriptyline and desipramine are often used because of their lower rate of the anticholinergic side effects that might affect balance and safety. Effective dosage levels for older patients may be substantially lower than that for younger populations. The motto "start low, go slow" for medicine use to avoid side effects might be revised with the elderly patient to "start very, very low; go very, very slow."

MAO inhibitors were found to be comparatively effective in treating elderly patients (Georgotas, McCue, and Hapworth, 1986). Particularly if diet can be controlled, as it can be in a nursing home environment, and if regular monitoring for hypertensive problems can be done, these medicines may be useful. The new generation of MAO inhibitors, called the MAO-A medicines, which are available in Europe but not yet in the United States, may be helpful with depression yet without causing these diet- and hypertension-related side effects (Lecrubier and Guelfi, 1990).

Most frequently, and particularly for outpatients, the newer generation of selective serotonin reuptake inhibitors (SSRIs) are the medicines of choice. The shorter half-life of medicines such as Zoloft (sertraline) and Paxil (paroxetine) make them more suitable for elderly patients who are sensitive to side effects, which more quickly dissipate than in SSRIs with a longer half-life, such as Prozac (fluoxetine). Wellbutrin (bupropion) may be particularly useful with the elderly (Roose, Glassman, and Giardina, 1987). This medicine may be particularly indicated for patients with Parkinson's disease who are also depressed.

St. Dennis (1995) reports anecdotal evidence that Desyrel (trazodone) may help with depression in elderly patients with dementia. This very sedating drug may also help reduce aggressiveness in elderly patients. St. Dennis notes that trazodone may be the drug of choice to use with "screamers" in institutional settings, a benefit that would certainly warrant its consideration.

Augmenting medicines can be used, although the fragility of elderly patients and their vulnerability to side effects must be taken into account. Trazodone or one of the tricyclics is often given to enhance the effectiveness of the prescribed SSRI when the initial medicine alone is insufficient to remove the signs and symptoms of depression. It should be recalled that adding these medicines to the SSRI greatly increases their blood levels. Blood levels should be carefully monitored to avoid toxicity. BuSpar (buspirone) may enhance serotonin effectiveness with antidepressant medicines used by the elderly, and seems to have a very benign side-effect profile. This may be particularly indicated in elderly patients with concomitant anxiety. Some anecdotal reports suggest that the anxiolytic effect may not occur when the SSRI is combined with BuSpar, or may even have a paradoxical effect, but this has not been explored to date in research with the elderly. Electroconvulsive therapy can also be used quite successfully with the elderly (Hay, 1993).

Elderly patients are far more vulnerable to comorbidity with conditions that can affect therapeutic results of antidepressant medicines. Memory problems and a lack of support to enhance adherence may cause them to misuse or overuse other medicines as well as prescribed antidepressants. Alcohol abuse is a risk with the elderly, creating an increased likelihood of interaction between alcohol and medicines.

The psychosocial contributions to depression in the elderly cannot be ignored. One study, for example (Reynolds et al., 1992), showed that antidepressant medicines combined with interpersonal psychotherapy resulted in a very high—about 75%—treatment success rate. This program emphasized psychoeducational orientation and supportive treatment, as well as a focus on interpersonal factors that can affect depression, perhaps leading to a significant reduction in medical utilization.

There are a number of psychosocial factors that can increase risk for depression. Loneliness and isolation are high on the list. Elderly patients may have disruptions in support as a result of life transitions, decreased mobility, and reduced economic resources. Social programs for the elderly can provide an opportunity to rebuild ongoing social relationships. Church programs for seniors, elder hostel programs, organized travel for senior groups, and a variety of other resources may be helpful. Agencies that deal with aging and elderly populations provide a variety of specialized resources helpful in the adjunctive treatment of elderly patients. The reliance on external resources is important in managed care, and the therapist treating elderly patients needs to know about these resources.

10

Special Problems: Dual Diagnosis, Refractory Depression, and Suicide

DUAL DIAGNOSIS

Depression and other disorders of mood are usually discussed as if they occurred independently of other conditions or problems. Very often, however, depression coexists with other psychological or behavioral problems, which can obscure the diagnostic picture and complicate treatment planning. In reality, patients often present with many problems, of which depression may be but one. Although depression can coexist with any other nonmood disorder (unless precluded by the diagnostic definitions in *DSM-IV*; e.g., a major depressive disorder that might be better accounted for by the diagnosis of a schizoaffective disorder), there are some diagnoses which are seen more frequently with depression than others. Anxiety disorders, personality disorders (including obsessive-compulsive personality), somatization disorders, alcohol- and substance-use problems, and eating disorders are commonly seen in depressed patients. While a thorough discussion of these disorders is certainly beyond the scope of this book, we will review some of the more common ones as they affect depression and conclude with some thoughts about treatment approaches in dual diagnosis. In managed care, conditions may be treated sequentially, rather than simultaneously, for effective management of resources. Particular approaches for a patient with a dual diagnosis are appropriate.

Somatoform Disorders and Pain

DSM-IV includes a variety of diagnoses within the so-called "somatoform disorders," conditions in which physical, or somatic, symptoms are reflective of psychological rather than medical difficulties. In these conditions psychological factors may cause or exacerbate medical problems, cause them to have a greater than expected effect upon the patient's life, or cause a preoccupation with health that results in intensive use of health care resources. There are a variety of ways in which a diagnosis for a somatization disorder can be distinguished from a diagnosis for a depressive disorder in the diagnostic nomenclature. For example, somatization demands at least eight symptoms in four different symptom domains to justify the diagnosis, and symptom display must persist over a period of years. This frequency and intensity of physical symptoms exceed those of depressive disorders. Depression seems, however, to play a role in many somatic symptoms.

Katon, Kleinman, and Rosen (1982), reviewing research studies employing a variety of depression inventories, concluded that when depression is not self-reported in patients who present with somatic symptoms to their primary-care physician, the diagnosis of depression is missed more than 90% of the time. Conversely, Lindsay and Wyckoff (1981) showed that pain symptoms occurred in almost two thirds of medical patients with major depressive disorder. Numerous studies, with a total subject sample of almost 1,000 medical patients with depressive symptoms, show a high rate of significant pain complaints, ranging between 30 and 87% in the various studies (Katon, 1988; Large, 1986; Walker and Greene, 1989). Katon also estimates that between 12 and 35% of the patients in primary care in these studies were significantly depressed. Katon (1987) later suggested that 30-50% of those with some depressive signs and symptoms met the formal criteria for major depressive episodes.

One study (Dworkin, von Korff, and LeResche, 1990) found that

1,000 patients with a single pain complaint were no more depressed than controls. Katon (1987) found that patients with two or more pain complaints were six times more likely than controls to have clinical depression. The implication of these studies is that a majority of patients with depression have some pain complaints, and that treating the depression alleviates the pain.

There are various theories about this connection. One theory, which is supported by correlative data, is that the physical symptoms are brought about by the underlying condition of a major depressive disorder. Another somewhat more subtle theory seems better to fit other evidence of the prevalence of somatic symptoms. About 80% of healthy individuals experience some somatic symptoms in any one week (Katon, 1991). Katon (1995) reports that community studies reveal an average of a new symptom every 5 to 7 days, but 95% of people don't see a physician. Studies of the general population show that fully 20% have fatigue symptoms (Katon, 1995). Katon focuses on the maintenance and social definition of pain rather than its causes, suggesting that depression lowers the threshold at which a person perceives minor symptoms and considers them to require medical attention.

An analogy might be that of a fairly large lake which is artificially lowered each year in order to control runoff over the dams. When the water level is high, sandbars close to the surface are submerged. As the water level lowers, islands form. The lowering of the water level, not the nature of the sandbars, which are fairly consistent, determines the presence of the islands. This analogy suggests that psychosocial stress "lowers the water level" of a patient's emotional reserves and causes somatic symptoms—at other times overlooked or considered irrelevant—to be more obvious to the patient and to prompt help-seeking behavior. Other theories of somatization would suggest that depression may determine both the *presence* of some of the sandbars and their *visibility* as islands when they rise above the surface.

Both theories have much apparent utility and relevance. Jenkins, Kleinman, and Good (1991), in a cross-cultural study of depression, noted that Western psychiatry tends to emphasize a mood-based definition of depression, while in many nonwestern societies depression is expressed in the idiom of bodily complaints. Kirmayer

(1987) discusses somatization as both a sociolinguistic *and* a psycho-physiological process.

Whatever the connection, depression seems to cause complaints of physical symptoms and to prompt their medical evaluation. Conversely, medical illness or physical symptoms can also cause a loss or lack of significant rewards or satisfactions in life and lead to depression. An exacerbation of depressive problems stemming from, rather than causing, pain symptoms may also be a component of this.

Fibromyalgia

Kellner (1991) discusses the complex interaction among fibromyalgia and other myofacial pain syndromes. Muscular aches and pains are the presenting symptoms of fibromyalgia, a common complaint seen by physicians specializing in rheumatology. It can occur with varying degrees of severity and a range of symptoms, although characteristic symptoms include multiple and widespread "tender points," sleep disorders, and complaints of swelling and numbness. Kellner notes that in some patients fibromyalgia may have a physical display in tissue pathology, but the nature and extent of this are still not fully understood. He suggests that a chain of factors—including physical disease, disorders of mood, and other psychological problems initially causing sleep difficulties, which reduce pain threshold—can culminate in complaints of fibromyalgia. It has been suggested that depression may often play a role in fibromyalgia, but the relationship is very controversial and apparently complex. Hudson, Hudson, Pliner, Goldenberg, and Pope (1985) found that 72% of a small sample of patients with fibromyalgia had either current or past depression. Given that sleep disruptions can accompany depression and can affect physical well-being in a variety of ways, this correlation cannot be used to prove causation.

Chronic Fatigue

Chronic fatigue can be either a symptom or a syndrome qualifying for a diagnosis. As a symptom it refers merely to a pervasive feeling of being tired. As a syndrome it refers to a chronic and recurrent debilitating fatigue, which may be accompanied by weakness, fever, difficulties in concentration, and depressive symptoms. There is much mystery about the cause of this condition, and some even question its existence and find it hard to distinguish chronic fatigue from depressive or somatization disorders. Still, it is a frequent complaint.

The etiology of chronic fatigue syndrome may be less relevant to treatment than one would think. Although some patients with chronic fatigue appear to have an immunological complication from a previous viral infection, responsive antiviral agents have not proven helpful in the treatment of chronic fatigue, nor has any medical treatment been found to be particularly effective. Rehabilitation programs in which patients with chronic fatigue are encouraged gradually to increase the amount of physical activity, to set realistic goals, to increase their perception of control over symptoms, and to engage in systematic exercise have been effective. These are many of the same behavioral approaches that help with depression, suggesting that even if chronic fatigue stems from a medical cause, such as the residual effects of a viral infection, the diagnosis and treatment of a depressive disorder may be helpful.

It is also of interest that the signs and symptoms associated with depression may also affect immune competency (Glaser et al., 1985; Locke et al., 1984). Stress, particularly loneliness, can affect health. A lack of social integration combined with loneliness, as found in depression, may make one more vulnerable to a variety of medical conditions (Dalkvist, Wahlin, Bartsch, and Forsbeck, 1995).

Somatization

Somatization disorders have been found to correlate with a number of variables. Sifneos (1973) coined the term "alexithymia," which means "no words for mood," to describe the characteristic difficulty patients with psychosomatic disorders have expressing their emotions and moods. Other authors, for example Pennebaker (1985), suggest that repression, denial, or a failure to confide about distressing events and emotions may lead to somatization disorders. Pennebaker and O'Heeron (1984) found that among subjects whose spouses had died unexpectedly, the more they talked with others about their loss, the fewer physical symptoms they experienced and the healthier they reported feeling. The capacity to relate to other people on a direct and emotional level is an important component to preventing somatization. This also seems an important component in preventing somatization disorders and may also help to prevent depression.

Treatment with antidepressant medicines helps some patients with pain complaints. Some antidepressants, particularly amitriptyline, seem to have an analgesic effect on some forms of chronic pain. Onghena, DeCuyper, VanHoudenhove, and Verstraeten (1993) find very low-dose use of certain tricyclics to be more effective than placebos in treatment of some patients with chronic pain. They conclude that the analgesic effect is likely to be separate from the antidepressant effect, particularly given the very low levels at which these medicines are used and the finding that not all antidepressants have similar effectiveness. The association is intriguing in view of the data on pain symptoms and depression reported by Katon, who recommends that any primary care physician evaluating a patient with two or more unexplained pain complaints should be highly suspicious of major depressive disorder, since this is likely to be an accurate diagnosis.

Although somatization and depressive disorders are distinct categories in the diagnostic nomenclature, they do seem to overlap, and there are strong suggestions that depression is an important component for many who have somatic symptoms. Talley (1994) notes that the most common complaint of patients on the primary care level, who were later diagnosed as depressed, is not depression but fatigue. The majority of patients with depression also have some physical pain.

As noted, depression is often overlooked on the primary care level, both by patients and by their physicians. Being attentive to the role of depression in the very large population of depressed patients who use medical resources and treating depression effectively can result in great benefits to patients who may be suffering without appropriate care. Patients who are inappropriately diagnosed and treated may also be reinforced in their hypochondriacal concerns and mistake their problems as exclusively physical, rather than at least partially psychological, in origin. Further, the economic benefits of treating such patients effectively more than justify the cost of psychotherapy to the managed care organization. The research supports simultaneously responding to the somatization and depressive problems by treating the depression as a primary focus of care, at least with some patients and particularly with the elderly. With somatization disorder, treating the more debilitating depressive symptoms first seems appropriate, since physical symptoms may change after effective treatment.

Alcohol and Substance Abuse

Assessing the role of alcohol and substance abuse is important when treating any psychiatric condition, but particularly with mood disorders. Alcohol abuse is more common than alcohol dependence, but studies of those with the formal diagnosis of alcoholism provide information about patterns of alcohol use in mood disorders. The epidemiological catchment area study found a prevalence of alcoholism of approximately 5% (Helzer and Pryzbeck, 1988). This study also found that people who met the criteria for alcoholism were nearly twice as likely also to have a major depressive disorder.

It should be remembered that the conditions of depression and alcoholism are very distinct and do not reflect the same underlying condition, although they may be associated. Most studies have found that alcoholism is an unlikely outcome of depression (Deykin, Levy, and Wells, 1987; Hasin and Grant, 1987). Many therapists believe that depressed people treat their depression with alcohol. Although research suggests that this is not true for men, some studies (Depression Guideline Panel, 1993) find that women who are alcoholic are more likely to have a preexisting disorder of mood. However, most of the research indicates that these are distinct conditions. Adoption studies confirm the independent transmission of depression and alcoholism. Goodwin and colleagues (1973), and Goodwin, Schulsinger, Knopf, Mednick, and Guze (1977) found that sons and daughters of alcoholic parents were more likely to be alcoholic, but no more likely to be depressed.

The converse is not true, however. Although depressed people, or at least depressed males, are no more likely than nondepressed people to become alcoholic, alcoholics are much more likely to be depressed than nonalcoholics. Petty's (1992) review of 24 studies provides support for this view. Most of the studies show that between 10% and 30% of patients with alcoholism also suffer from depression. Four studies suggest that patients submitting to alcoholism treatment programs who are also depressed become less depressed during the first 2 to 4 weeks of sobriety (see, for example, Brown and Schuckit, 1988). Some studies find that patients who are both depressed and alcoholic on initial assessment were more likely to remain alcoholic than alcoholics who were not also depressed (Loosen, Dew, and Prange, 1990). However, a long follow-up study by O'Sullivan and colleagues (1988) finds no difference in outcome between patients with a dual diagnosis (alcoholism and depressive disorders) than in those who are only alcoholic.

In a study of 371 psychiatric admissions, Bernadt and Murray (1986) evaluated the history of drinking behavior, relating it to psychiatric diagnoses. They examined whether subjects with certain psychiatric disorders drank more heavily as their conditions worsened before admission to a hospital and found that drinking was not particularly associated with severity of mood disorder. Only those diagnosed as alcoholic drank more than average before requiring hospital-level care. Although some patients with bipolar disorder drank more, about the same percentage drank less during the month before admission. Ewusi-Mensah, Saunders, Wodak, Murray, and Williams (1983) also noted a lower rate of mood disorders among alcoholics in a liver treatment unit than in a psychiatric hospital, suggesting that there may be bias due to sample selection in some studies. Depressive disorders and alcoholism may be even less closely associated than the research on an unrepresentative sample of alcoholics patients in psychiatric hospitals might suggest.

The available data indicate that it is a mistake to view alcoholism as merely a symptom of "masked depression," and that the therapist should instead regard alcoholism as a separate syndrome that may contribute to depression, either behaviorally or biochemically. Although women may be more likely to use alcohol in an attempt to self-medicate for depressive symptoms, and are therefore at greater risk for alcoholism, it still seems that the patient with a dual diagnosis requires initial treatment for the alcohol abuse. After the patient stops drinking and is detoxified, treatment for any residual depression symptoms may proceed.

Other Substances

Kendall and Clarkin (1992), in a review of comorbidity and substance abuse, find that 32% of those with a mood disorder abuse substances, including alcohol and prescription medicines. As discussed in the section on children and adolescents, comorbidity of substance abuse and depression may be the rule rather than the exception, particularly for adolescents (see e.g., Lewinsohn, Hops, Roberts, Seeley, and Andrews, 1993).

The range of drugs abused, including prescription medicines used other than as prescribed and illegal drugs used in a variety of ways, makes it difficult to generalize about their effects on mood disorders. Some psychoactive agents can cause dysphoric mood and even suicidal thoughts. Some stimulants can create manic symptoms, or can cause depressive symptoms upon withdrawal. Length of use, extent of use, and the agent used can all determine the effects on mood disorders. For example, the relationship between cocaine and mood disorders is quite complex. Some studies show that use of antidepressants tends to reduce the relapse rate in cocaine users while others suggest that cocaine use may be correlated with a switch from unipolarity to bipolarity of mood disorder or with rapid cycling disorders. An assessment of substance use is important for a host of both diagnostic and dispositional reasons. The variability of effects on the neurochemistry of the brain from different drugs and from the varying purity of particular street drugs, makes any generalization about treatment impossible. Still, it makes sense to follow the paradigm useful in the treatment of alcoholism, responding to the substance problem first, and any residual depressive problem afterward.

Personality Disorders

Personality disorders are quite common among psychiatric patients, with most studies showing between 45% and 65% of those receiving treatment to have a personality disorder, as either a primary or a secondary condition (Depression Guideline Panel, 1993). Kendall and Clarkin (1992) estimate that 30 to 40% of depressed patients have comorbid personality disorders.

Personality disorders, much like substance-related disorders, are wide-ranging in their symptoms. The term "personality disorder" may refer to some behavioral patterns that could be the opposite of others similarly diagnosed. *DSM-IV* clusters these personality disorders into three groups. Cluster A refers to disorders which can be characterized as odd, such as paranoid, schizoid, or schizotypal disorders. Cluster B diagnoses are used for disorders which express themselves in overly dramatic, overly emotional, or erratic behavior, such as the antisocial, histrionic, borderline or narcissistic personality disorders. Cluster C includes those disorders that are characterized as anxious, fearful, and timid, such as the avoidant, obsessive-compulsive, dependent, and passive-aggressive personality disorders. All of these conditions may coexist with depression, though it may be that the cluster C disorders behaviorally predispose affected people to depressive problems.

Many studies examine patients with both personality and major depressive disorders (Shea, Glass, Pilkonis, Watkins, and Docherty, 1987; Black, Bell, Hulbert, and Nasrallah, 1988). These studies generally show that a personality disorder complicates treatment and prognosis. Those with personality disorders tended to have earlier-onset depressions, to experience more frequent and longer depressive episodes with more severe symptoms, and to respond less well to antidepressant medicines and psychotherapy, experiencing more symptomatology on follow-up. These studies also found increased rates of suicide attempts and self-harm, particularly among patients with a borderline personality disorder.

The incidence of false positive diagnoses of personality disorders is higher when a major depressive disorder is also present (see Oldham et al., 1992). This suggests that diagnosis of a personality disorder might best be considered somewhat tentative if it coexists with depression, since a symptom display of an apparent personality disorder might change after treatment for depression. Those who were diagnosed with a personality disorder well before a depressive episode, increasing the likelihood of an enduring behavioral pattern separate from depressive symptoms, were found to respond more slowly to treatment, to have more complex histories, and to exhibit greater disturbance in social functioning. They may still improve with treatment, however. Frank and colleagues (1990) found that a significant portion of their patients who might have been labeled "refractory" or "treatment resistant" after eight weeks ultimately responded to treatment with medicines and improved with continuing treatment. These data indicate that patients with both personality and depressive disorders should be treated primarily for the depression, and assessed for a personality disorder after depressive symptoms have abated. A personality disorder should be nonprovisionally diagnosed only after treatment for depression.

Of course, those who treat such patients need to take into account the effect of personality disorders on the consistency of treatment, adherence to medication regimens, candor, and cooperativeness. It is the consideration of the unique personality and goal structure of each patient that makes psychotherapy an art, whether these personality patterns are within the normal range or are so problematic as to qualify for a diagnosis of personality disorder. Treatment strategy is different from treatment target, and the best approach appears to focus on the depressive symptoms rather than the personality disorder symptoms if a clear-cut diagnosis exists. An exception to this might be the borderline personality disorder, discussed in Linehan (1993). The patient with this disorder requires special consideration with respect to treatment, particularly regarding the use of medicines. The suicidal and parasuicidal behavior which characterizes this disorder mandates a different response.

Eating Disorders

Eating disorders include anorexia nervosa and bulimia nervosa. Anorexia is defined as refusal to maintain body weight over a minimal normal level, combined with other signs and symptoms such as a fear of becoming fat, disturbance of body image, and sometimes amenorrhea. Anorexia is found quite often in younger populations, perhaps in as many as 0.2% to 0.8% of adolescent girls, compared to .05% to 0.1% of adults in community samples (Robins et al., 1984). Bulimia is characterized by binge eating, the rapid consumption of large amounts of food. There is common use of vomiting, laxatives, or other means to control weight after the eating episodes, by which the patient makes up for a loss of self-control. Up to 1% of adolescents and young women may experience this, although rates of up to 22% in some age groups have been found in studies of those seen in the primary care settings (Robins et al., 1984).

There are no large studies of the prevalence of eating disorders among patients with major depressive disorder but it has been well established that many patients with eating disorders are also depressed. The Depression Guideline Panels estimate from reviews of studies that between 50 and 75% of patients with eating disorders have a lifetime history of major depressive disorder (Depression Guideline Panel, 1993).

Undernutrition is frequently seen in eating disorders, and this may bring about depressive symptoms. Sleep problems, cognitive difficulties, and irritability are all physical consequences of eating disorders. These symptoms which appear depressive may subside when better nutrition and a healthy weight level have been reestablished, indicating that treatment for an eating disorder should probably focus first on the eating disorder itself, rather than any associated depression. Although antidepressants may be used as a mechanism to control the eating disorder problems (e.g., Pope, Hudson, Jonas, and Yurgelun-Todd, 1983), the treatment program best targets the symptoms of the eating disorder rather than the underlying causes. Cognitive behavioral therapy is very useful with this disease (Ballenger, 1994). Given the medical dangers accompanying eating disorders, in both the short and the long term, as well as the potential lethality of these conditions, coordinated and effective treatment is essential. Treatment for depression can occur following a resurrection of normal eating patterns, should the depression persist.

Anxiety Disorders

Depressive symptoms and anxiety symptoms frequently coexist. Community studies show a very high rate of comorbidity. About

30% of outpatients with major depressive disorder also meet the criteria for generalized anxiety disorder at some time during the course of their illness. In about half of these the general anxiety disorder preceded the major depressive disorder. Panic disorder has been found in almost 20% of those with a major depression in the ECA data, and one study even found 91% of patients with agoraphobia developed a mood disorder over a three-year follow-up (Munjack and Moss, 1981; Angst and Dobler-Mikola, 1985).

As noted in the discussion on theories of depression, some even see the overlap between anxiety and depression as so significant to indicate they are actually a single condition, that of Negative Emotion (N.E.), though with different displays. The decision about which disorder to treat first may depend upon which sign and symptom complex begins first, which is the most incapacitating, which is the most pronounced in a family history, and which the patient most wishes to address.

It should be recalled that anxiety disorders may augment suicidal risk. The rate of suicide attempts for persons with both panic and major depressive disorders is twice that for those with panic disorders alone, almost 20% over the course of a lifetime (Johnson, Weissman, and Klerman, 1990). Both disorders separately are associated with suicide rates, as noted by Coryell, Noyes, and Clancy (1982).

Obsessive–Compulsive Disorders

Obsessive-compulsive disorders (OCD) tend to overlap with depression. The Depression Guidelines Panel (1993) notes that most studies show a lifetime occurrence of depressive symptoms in those with OCD as high as 80% to even 100%, even though only about 10–30% of OCD patients meet the criteria for major depressive disorder at any one time. Goodwin and Jamison (1990) reviewed 13 follow-up studies and found that major depression tended to occur after OCD.

It has also been noted that patients with OCD are likely to have a family history of depression. In the ECA data analysis, OCD symptoms were found in a third of those with major depression and in 15% of those with dysthymia. It is important to make a good diagnosis of OCD, since severe depression may have obsessive and ruminative features, different from "true OCD." Compulsions are usually lacking, but recurrent ruminations may be present, with the depressed patient. These ruminations are usually about negative events, negative self-perceptions, or guilty preoccupations. These patients do not meet the criteria for OCD, but may instead have severe or even recurrent depressive disorders.

The question may be somewhat moot, however. OCD is increasingly treated with medicines, including the SSRIs. One such medicine, Luvox (fluvoxamine), is even used as an antidepressant in Europe, but marketed as a medicine for OCD in the United States. Prozac (fluoxetine) is approved for treatment of both depression and OCD. It is not surprising that treatment employing medication for OCD often results in the lessening of depressive symptoms, since antidepressant medicines are frequently used in these treatment programs. As with depression and comorbid panic disorder, OCD is more effectively treated over the long term with a treatment program that includes behavioral and cognitive behavioral therapy. Signs and symptoms of OCD improve in about 60% of the patients using medicines alone; however, the relapse rate is 90[+]% when the medication is withdrawn. This relapse rate is very low when psychotherapy is used (Swinson, 1994).

If OCD is present to a degree to warrant a separate diagnosis, it should be treated first. If depression merely results in some symptoms of OCD short of a formal diagnosis, the depression should be treated first.

Other Mood Disorders

Finally, it should be recalled that a major depressive disorder can coexist with other mood disorders, particularly dysthymic disorders. One can receive the diagnosis of both dysthymic and major depressive disorders, or "double depression," as it is sometimes called. The ECA studies (Weissman and Myers, 1978), reanalyzed by the Depression Guideline Panel (1993), showed that for patients with a dysthymic disorder, reexamination a year later found that 10% had a major depressive disorder, between 5 and 20% had both, between 11% and 23% had some other depressive problem, and perhaps less than a quarter still had dysthymic disorder. The *DSM-IV* notes that if a dysthymic disorder precedes the onset of a major depressive disorder, there is less likelihood of a full spontaneous interepisode recovery between major depressive episodes and greater likelihood of more frequent episodes in recurrent depressive disorders. It is also noted that dysthymic disorder is more common among first-degree biological relatives of people with major depression among the general population.

The severe, debilitating, and sometimes psychotic features of a major depressive disorder require initial treatment, with follow-up treatment for the underlying dysthymia. Continued treatment can address the impairments, dysfunction, and dissatisfaction caused by dysthymia, and can reduce the risk for recurrent depressions.

REFRACTORY DEPRESSION

Some cases of depressive disorders don't get better with treatment. These conditions are called refractory disorders. Nonresponse to treatment is usually indicated by incomplete or no response during the acute phase of treatment, no response to maintenance treatment, or relapse during the maintenance phase (Gerner, 1994). Failure to respond is characteristically noticed first during the acute management phase, and most discussions on treatment of refractory depression refers to those patients who don't get better, rather than to those who don't stay better or suffer relapse.

Major Depressive Disorder

Nonresponse is a common problem with biological treatments. With major depressive disorder no more than half the patients achieve the desired results from antidepressant medicines, although perhaps another quarter of treated patients gain some benefit short of what is sought (Nierenberg, 1995). A longer time response than expected often indicates a refractory depressive disorder, which requires a different approach.

This raises the question of how much time should pass before a course of biological treatment is declared less than optimally effective. The Depression Guideline Panel (1993) recommends that if by the end of six weeks, the patient has not responded to medication at all or with minimal symptomatic relief, two steps are necessary: (1) reassessment of the accuracy of the diagnosis; and (2) reassessment of the adequacy of the treatment. The guidelines also describe alternative approaches for patients with no significant response by the end of six weeks, or perhaps by the end of four weeks in the severely ill, including: continuing medication at an adjusted dosage, discontinuing the first medicine and beginning a second, adding an adjunctive treatment, perhaps augmenting with a second medicine or psychotherapy, and obtaining a referral.

Nierenberg (1995), director of the Depression Research Program at Massachusetts General Hospital in Boston, finds that a response to Prozac as early as two weeks into treatment tends to be predictive of future effectiveness, since there is less than a 40% chance of response by the end of eight weeks for those who do not respond earlier. He finds that if there is no response by week 4, there is less than a 20% chance of response after eight weeks. The chance of response declines to about 6% by week 8 if no response is seen by the sixth week. Nierenberg proposes that if there is no response to fluoxetine at the four- to six-week range, some change should be made. He concludes that raising the dosage or combining the Prozac with other medicines might be helpful. He discourages discontinuation of the medicine at this time, arguing that a longer trial of this medicine at an increased dosage or when augmented by others seems more appropriate.

With the older tricyclic antidepressants prescription at too low a dose to prove effective was one of the primary causes of inadequate response. As noted, many of these medicines were prescribed by primary care physicians. Further, side effects often prohibited patients to continue taking these medicines at a dosage that could produce a therapeutic response (Salzman, 1993).

With the tricyclics, increasing dosages up to the maximum level recommended by the Physician's Desk Reference (PDR) is often effective. Following that, accurately diagnosed major depressive disorder patients able to tolerate side effects might even warrant referral to a university department of psychiatry for consideration of treatment above dosage levels normally recommended.

With the newer medicines it is somewhat easier to determine appropriate dosages for treatment, in contrast with the older tricyclic medicines, with which blood levels had to be evaluated in order to establish that a patient was receiving too little or too much of the medicine or taking it at all. With the SSRIs the standard dosage is narrower. Approximately 85% of patients respond to 50–100 mg a day of (Zoloft) sertraline, and to 20 mg a day of (Paxil) paroxetine or Prozac (Salzman, 1993). Although higher dosages may be very helpful for some, the vast majority of patients will either respond to a standard dosage or will not respond at all, and this is apparent comparatively early on. Fava and colleagues (1994) compared the effects of doubling the dosage of Prozac from 20 to 40 mg a day to augmenting it with other medicines. They found that the dosage increase is sometimes superior to augmentation although augmentation is also often helpful.

Lithium sometimes is employed to augment SSRIs or TCAs. Ontiveros, Fontaine, and Elie (1991) compared augmentation with lithium in desipramine and fluoxetine and found improvement in almost two thirds of the patients in each group. Those taking the Prozac responded more quickly, usually within the first two weeks. Similar results have been found by Katona (1993).

Other drug combinations are sometimes used. BuSpar (Buspirone) is an antianxiety agent increasingly popular for augmentation of SSRIs. Nierenberg (1995) believes that, despite the lack of controlled trials, case studies support its use.

Tricyclic medicines can be added to SSRIs, though at much lower dosages. Salzman (1993) warns that tricyclic dosages must be very low since the SSRIs can raise blood levels of tricyclics to toxic levels. He proposes, for example, use of 25 mg of desipramine or even 10 mg of nortriptyline to avoid toxicity. It is quite common to prescribe 100 mg of a tricyclic along with 20 mg of Prozac. Case reports suggest the blood levels of the Prozac may be boosted fourfold by the tricyclic but there are no controlled studies of this to date. The increased risk of serotonin syndrome in augmentation therapies, though low, is something that even nonmedical therapists need to watch for, since they are most likely to monitor patients in ongoing treatment.

Use of thyroid medicines has been found helpful as an augmentation strategy with both tricyclics and SSRIs. Joffe, Levitt, Bagby, MacDonald, and Singer (1993) found that augmentation of tricyclics with lithium and with thyroid had equivalent outcomes, both being effective in about 60% of patients in acute care.

Stimulants, including Ritalin (methylphenidate), Cylert (pemoline), and even certain amphetamines, are sometimes used in treatment for depression. Although some research has found stimulants helpful, few controlled studies have been done. Nierenberg (1995) points out the comorbidity of attention-deficit/hyperactivity disorder (ADHD) with depression, perhaps as high as 8% of outpatients, according to strict criteria. He has found no difference between subjects with and without ADHD with respect to onset, chronicity, duration, or response to medicines. It may be, however, that medicines used for ADHD help with an aspect of behavioral or cognitive limitation associated with depression. Such medicine augmentation, however, should be left to specialists in psychopharmacology. The risk of misuse of these medicines and legal standards may require rigorous justification for their continued prescription.

It should also be noted that some augmentation strategies can be dangerous. MAO inhibitors, for example, can be harmful, or even lethal, if used concomitantly with SSRIs. In fact, a long "wash-out" of many weeks is recommended before initiating MAO treatment following the use of an SSRI.

Substitutions of medicines are sometimes indicated. The fact that a patient has not responded to one medicine does not predict nonresponsiveness to other medicines in a correctly diagnosed major depressive disorder. Even among the SSRIs, nonresponsiveness to one does not predict nonresponsiveness to another. Substituting one medicine for another in a slightly different class is perhaps more common, however, and it makes intuitive sense. For example, Effexor (venlafaxine) is often employed as a substitute when an SSRI has been found to be ineffective.

Bipolar Disorders

Use of lithium carbonate alone was once regarded as adequate treatment for the vast majority of patients diagnosed with a bipolar disorder. Sachs (1995) notes that many of the research studies of lithium treatment are rigorously controlled, with patients carefully selected for a single diagnosis of manic depressive illness. This seems to be a very unrepresentative sample, however, particularly in those studies which exclude patients with substance abuse or alcohol-related problems, since up to two thirds of the patients with a diagnosis of bipolar disorder also have these additional problems. It is estimated that up to 65% also have some anxiety-related difficulties (Sachs, 1995). Considering that those patients with multiple diagnoses and substance-related problems are more inclined to come into a clinic, only about a third of all patients with a bipolar disorder are eligible for participation in the more rigorous studies. Sachs studied the larger, more representative population of outpatients with bipolar disorder, those who had multiple diagnoses and problems, and found that only 4% of those patients on lithium alone stayed well through the year. Sachs estimates that perhaps 90% of patients with bipolar disorders involving more than three manic episodes, who are treated with lithium alone, fail to adequately respond.

With bipolar disorders it is possible to change or augment medicines, but discontinuing lithium should only be done cautiously. Goodwin (1994) notes that "the worst mistake you can make is to take a person off lithium" inappropriately. As mentioned earlier, discontinuation of lithium can cause later nonresponsiveness to the drug. Poor compliance or mistaken prescription habits may cause refractory bipolar disorders in patients formerly treatable with maintenance dosages of this medicine. As Sachs (1995) notes, "the indication to stop treatment has to be something other than the fact that treatment has worked." There may also be significant risk of relapse if lithium is discontinued. Goodwin (1994) proposes discussing the question of discontinuation with the family and comparing the risk of mania to the risk of maintaining the patient without medicine.

There are other causes of nonresponsiveness to lithium. Psychotic symptoms, alcohol and substance abuse, severity of mania, and the presence of mixed mood episodes make response to lithium less likely (Sachs, 1995).

Adding medicines is often the first consideration with refractory bipolar disorders. Goodwin (1994) notes that in most studies of use of anticonvulsants, at least with carbamazepine, lithium is also given. Gerner (1994), however, suggests first switching to anticonvulsants with patients who are nonresponsive to lithium, then switching anticonvulsants, and finally attempting polypharmacy.

There are many theories about the use of medications in bipolar disorders, and these are likely to change. It has been suggested that MAO inhibitors may be helpful adjuncts to treatment. New MAO inhibitors, available in Europe, do not require the dietary changes necessitated by the use of those currently available in the United States. Specialists who are knowledgeable about drug interactions, familiar with new interventions, and attentive to the risk and benefits of augmenting and substituting various agents should be consulted, most particularly with refractory cases of bipolar disorders. In a managed care context, however, it is likely that such specialists will serve by referral rather than as primary mental health providers.

The person making the primary intervention will still play a vital role in treatment. Continuation treatment and effective management of care seem especially vital for patients with bipolar disorder. Lithium is still the primary intervention for bipolar disorders. A UCLA study reported by Gerner (1994) showed that only 20–50% of patients adhered to ongoing medicine maintenance with lithium, largely because of the side effects. Behavioral techniques to enhance adherence, discussed in the chapter on treatment of major mood disorders, seem particularly important.

It is important to do a thorough and complete assessment of patients presenting with symptoms of bipolar disorders. A good history is necessary when considering alternative responses to refractory mood disorders, and a helpful diagnosis will include information about length of cycles, severity of cycles, and presence of depressive symptoms. Nierenberg (1995) also points out that severity of depression is greatest in many patients during manic episodes, and that the mean Hamilton depression score is highest for patients with mixed bipolar symptoms during their manic phases. He also notes that asking a patient about mania often produces poor data, since patients may not see the manic state as undesirable, atypical, or remarkable, and they may describe only depressive symptoms on intake. Failure to inquire more closely, reliance on verbal report rather than inquiring about behavioral indicia of mania, or failure to use ancillary resources may cause the clinician to "miss the mark." In this case, the clinician is likely to prescribe an antidepressant medicine, which may trigger a bipolar disorder and consequently enhance refractoriness.

Other Treatment Considerations

Mood disorders may not respond to treatment, but it is more difficult to gauge whether nonbiological treatment is working than it is to evaluate the effectiveness of medicines or of ECT. Assessing specific signs and symptoms and targeting outcomes may help in the evaluation of treatment effectiveness and almost certainly will be a component of managed care.

With those patients for whom an adequate trial of a proven clinical intervention is not helpful, it makes sense to consider changing therapeutic modes, much as one might consider changing medicines in the major mood disorders. One can augment nonbiological treatment with additional therapy, such as group therapy or psychoeducational classes. As with medicines, specific treatments can also be changed. We find it particularly helpful to consider changing one's level of system response and exploring whether family or social system factors may inhibit or preclude individual patient response. At a bare minimum, refractoriness suggests the need to involve others, who are significant in a patient's life, in treatment, either for gathering information or for exploring more potent treatment interventions by expanding the "treatment team." Well-formed interventions, demonstrated by the research to be effective, which fail to produce results strongly suggest family system or social system dysfunctions, and may indicate the need for different treatment.

Finally, if alternatives have been explored and treatment is not working, it seems valid to stop treatment. A therapist in managed care must come to terms with limits, and there are limits to the effectiveness of mental health interventions. Although we used to think that all patients with bipolar disorders responded to lithium and that depressed patients all got better with use of antidepressants, this is clearly not the case. A majority of patients fail to show significant recovery from these interventions so hopefully viewed in the past. Although psychotherapy has demonstrated its effectiveness in some disorders, it is not a "cure-all" and is not treatment of choice in severe and psychotic disorders. There is a high rate of recurrence of mood episodes even after electroconvulsive therapy. Patients with personality disorders are quite refractory to care, and some personality disorders may interact with depressive symptoms and syndromes. In other words, there may be some people we can't help, even with all of our horses hitched to the treatment wagon.

A danger in managed care is reaching this conclusion too quickly. Refractoriness cannot be assumed merely on the basis of simple rules, such as nonresponsiveness to medicines at 6 weeks. A significant portion of patients do respond to changes in medicine regimens subsequently, and an 8- to 12-week trial of antidepressants may be necessary before treatment failure can be declared, particularly in patients with coexisting personality disorders (Salzman, 1993). In the less evolved managed care systems which authorize a fixed number of sessions for patients, regardless of recurrence, comorbidity, severity, or medicine responsiveness, the limitations on duration of treatment need to be carefully considered in treatment planning. A patient with a severe bipolar problem which will pose chronic difficulties requires that therapy be rationed. More intensive involvement initially may ensure an accurate diagnosis, enhance the likelihood of adherence to prescription regimens, and involve family members in obtaining reliable reports of treatment effects. Then, however, it might be prudent to carefully ration the limited remaining sessions. This way the effects of medicine can be monitored, and the almost certain use of polypharmacy approaches can be explored with perhaps fewer sessions spread over a longer period of time, allowing better assessment of and adjustment to medicines.

It is the refractory and recurrent conditions that seem to pose the greatest challenge for managed care organizations. One hopes that managed care approaches will become sufficiently evolved, sophisticated, and humane that treatment of those with refractory depressions is a relevant concern. These patients are more at risk for suicide, require more hospital care, and have greater social impairment, all of which translate into higher costs. A sophisticated program will respond to refractory depressive disorders, with knowledgeable appraisal and algorithms for intervention which allow such patients to receive appropriate care rather than to be prematurely terminated.

There may be some patients whom we cannot help, but deliberate treatment is most likely to be efficient in taking care of them, particularly when compared with nonmanaged and more meandering intervention approaches. One hopes that managed care will address the needs of this patient population and avoid limiting resources to the point that refractory depression, which could be effectively treated, remains refractory.

SUICIDE

Suicide is a risk for depressed patients. The data regarding the magnitude of that risk can be viewed in either reassuring or alarming ways. On the one hand, suicide accounts for 25,000 deaths each year in the United States. Rates of suicide are increasing in children, and suicide is now the second most common cause of death among young people age 15–24 years of age (OPCS, 1990). Shaffer (1988) notes that the rate has doubled among white males aged 15–19, from 8 per 100,000 in the 1960s to almost 16 per 100,000 in the mid-1980s. About one adolescent every 90 minutes commits suicide. Some follow-up studies of depressed patients have reported that about one in six die by suicide. Although Roy (1994) notes that many of these studies were carried out before medicinal prophylaxis was available, Goodwin and Jamison (1990) reviewed numerous later studies of patients with manic depressive disorders in a total population of more than 9,000. Of those who died, almost 20% died by suicide.

On the other hand, suicide accounts for, on the average, between 12 and 17 out of every 100,000 deaths in the United States each year. Suicide is a fairly low probability event. Most patients do not kill themselves. The vast majority of depressed patients never attempt to do so.

Nevertheless, it is a risk, and certainly depressed people show an elevated risk for suicide as compared to the general population. When diagnosis is factored into the equation, those with a diagnosis of either a major mood disorder or dysthymic disorder are estimated to have a higher prevalence rate for suicide, almost 600 per 100,000 for male patients and perhaps 250 per 100,000 for female patients (Roy, 1994).

Parasuicide, Violence, and Suicide

Related to suicide is what is called "parasuicide." Kreitman (1977) defines it as behaviors which are nonfatal but intentionally self-injurious and which result in actual tissue damage, illness, or risk of death. He also uses this term for any injection of drugs or other substances other than as prescribed, if done with the intent to cause harm or death. Kreitman's criteria include suicide attempts and other self-injuries, including self-mutilations that are often a part of the diagnostic display of the borderline personality disorder. Intent seems important to qualify for the diagnosis of parasuicide as Kreitman uses the term. Parasuicide does not result from mistaken attempts to gain relief, such as taking an overdose of sleeping pills to get to sleep. Suicide threats also do not fall under this definition unless self-damaging behavior accompanies the verbal threat. Changing one's thinking about suicide, or even putting oneself at risk and not completing the act, such as by loading a gun and pointing it at oneself, and then putting it down and unloading it, would also not be considered parasuicidal behavior.

The concept of parasuicide has evoked much interest. Van Egmond and Diekstra (1989) have proposed a somewhat different definition for nonfatal suicidal behaviors. They distinguish parasuicide from attempted suicide, and narrow the definition of parasuicide to include only acts that cause or could cause self-harm in order to "bring about desired changes in consciousness and/or social condition."

Those who have looked closely at the differences among attempted suicide, parasuicide, and suicide find it to be a less clear-cut distinction than one might wish. Cantor (1972) gives as an example the young man who stabbed himself, missing death by 1/16th of an inch. She sees luck and chance as making the distinctions in this case, not more notable psychological processes. She acknowledges the differences between these groups of behavior but believes the distinction might not be meaningful for a large percentage of people. There are demographic distinctions between groups of attempters versus completers. Cantor notes that the ratio of suicides committed by males to those committed by females is almost 5 to 1, but the ratio of males to females for attempted suicide is reversed. Even with these clear-cut differences, the argument is strong for viewing patients' suicidally related actions as individually meaningful regardless of lethality of outcome.

Much research on violence against others addresses an audience of those interested in criminal behavior, with research funded by and reported to a somewhat separate group from that more concerned with issues of depression. Of interest is a similarity between some of the risk factors in suicide and parasuicidal behavior—which can be viewed as violence against self and perhaps symbolically against others—as compared with violence—defined as actions against others which are symbolically self-directed. The McArthur Risk Assessment Study for Violence (Monahan and Steadman, 1994) focuses on dispositional factors, historical factors, contextual factors, and clinical factors. Dispositional and demographic factors include age, gender, personality, and cognitive limits and strengths. Historical factors include social history, work history, and a history of mental hospitalization or violence. Contextual factors include perceived stress, social support, and means for violence. Clinical factors are the mental health diagnoses, on both Axis I and Axis II dimensions, with particular attention to substance abuse.

Similarly, Linehan (1981) has studied parasuicidal behavior with a focus on environmental, demographic, and behavioral characteristics using a multidimensional framework which is quite compatible with those used in the McArthur studies. Further, the similarity between violence and particularly parasuicidal behavior seems quite high. For example, both violent and parasuicidal patients are more likely to be unmarried than married, show a decreasing prevalence with age, are often very angry and impulsive, have low social involvement and support, and are quite prone to drug and alcohol abuse. Although there are ethnic and gender differences between parasuicidal and suicidal behavior, the differences between parasuicidal and violent behavior are not great. Although males may more likely be violent than females, and females more at risk for parasuicidal acts, there is a remarkable overlap between violence and parasuicide. Both violent and suicidal patients have lower serotonin levels than the general population (Linnoila et al., 1983).

We focus more upon risk factors for suicide, acknowledging that some who attempt suicide and some with parasuicidal behaviors may have many of the same criteria as the suicidal patient. The suicidal group is well defined, and more research has been compiled on suicide than on other self-injurious behaviors.

Risk Factors

Suicide is clearly relevant to the treatment of depression. Some see suicide as the ultimate outcome of severe depression. Viewing the complexity of the matter, and the intriguing relationship between suicide and violence, the connection seems far less clear-cut than some might think. As discussed by Baumeister (1993):

> Does depression cause suicide? The question has been very important to psychology and large amounts of information have been collected. At present, the best available answer is "not really." That is, it is undeniably true that depressed people attempt suicide at much higher rates than nondepressed people. But the depression itself is apparently not responsible for the suicide. Two facts are particularly telling. First, the vast majority of depressed people never attempt to kill themselves, so it cannot be argued simply that depression causes suicide. Second, when measures of hopelessness are included, depression fails to predict suicide independently. Depression and hopelessness often go together, but it is the hopelessness, not the depression, that leads to suicide. (p. 259)

Hopelessness may, in fact, be a necessary but insufficient condition for many suicides. Even if this is present, however, many other factors must come into play to culminate in a suicide. One can imagine a patient, a male in his fifties who has been laid off from work. Job prospects are not numerous, particularly given his age and the limited resources he brings to the marketplace. Somewhat depressed a few years ago, he left his wife after a passionate affair with another woman. Soon after he is laid off, this woman leaves him, ending the relationship and increasing his financial instability. His children have been alienated from him since the divorce, and he has not maintained many of his former friendships while pursuing his romance. He goes out at night to console himself, stopping at a local tavern, where he drinks a few more beers than he should. The beers help with some of the physical pain that he experiences from advancing arthritis. As the evening wears on he notices that his former girlfriend, for whom he has left wife and family, has arrived with one of his best friends from years gone by, one who was recently promoted at work. He drives home angry and depressed. He pulls into the garage, chancing to notice the rifle left loaded there from a recent hunting trip.

Many predictive risk factors are present here. Some people in this scenario would commit suicide. Others would not. If the person were to kill himself, what would be *the* cause? Would it be the depression, the alcohol, the gun, the physical pain, or the anger? Many of these "causes" are transitory, others more enduring. The effects of alcohol could wear off, the situational stimulus of the gun would not be there if it had been properly put away, and the grief over a relationship ending might pass, yet the depression, the pain, and the patient's age and gender would all persist. Would the extreme risk for suicide continue were the patient to load the gun and point it at himself and then change his mind? Possibly. Many who complete suicide have made a previous attempt, yet the majority of people who attempt suicide do not, in fact, later come to kill themselves.

There do seem to be some predisposing and precipitating factors. Predisposing factors include gender. More males kill themselves than females. More black adolescent males than white adolescent males commit suicide. A history of prior attempt increases risk for a future attempt and success. A family history of attempted suicide, suicide, or violence also seems to be a predictor. *Any* psychiatric hospitalization increases the risk for suicide, even if the hospitalization has not been for depression. The chronically mentally ill are more at risk for suicide than the general population. Witnessing a suicide has also been found to result in increased risk of suicide. Certain diagnoses seem overrepresented in suicide and completed suicides. For example, bipolar disorder, depressive disorder, alcoholism, and other drug addictions are found in greater numbers in suicidal populations than in the general population. A large body of research implicates anxiety, particularly panic episodes, as similarly overrepresented in the histories of those who commit suicide. Chronic pain may also predispose one to suicide.

Some personality factors seem to place one more at risk. A person who is perfectionistic or cognitively rigid may be less able to weather the storms of change and disappointment. A history of inadequate treatment may predispose one to future depression, increasing the risk for suicide. Limited treatment for recurrent depressions, or discontinuation of antidepressants short of the duration recommended by current research, are certainly relevant issues for managed care in that they may cause a person to be at greater risk for suicide. Biochemical factors may create a risk, with changes in 5-hydroxyindoleacetic acid in cerebral spinal fluid appearing in those who have completed suicide, a finding also reported in some studies of violence (Linnoila et al., 1983).

Among the precipitating factors, drinking is found to be an important correlate with suicide. A high percentage of those who commit suicide have been recently drinking and are intoxicated at the time of the suicide. Alcohol serves as a disinhibitant, provides emotional numbing to the magnitude or implications of one's actions, and may decrease available cognitive resources useful in arguing oneself away from suicidal thoughts and activities.

Baumeister (1993) points out that disappointment is a vital part of depression. He sees depression as stemming not so much from austerity or adversity as from a loss of previously favorable circumstances. Having it bad may not lead to suicide as much as having it *become* bad may predict suicide risk. He notes that suicide is more frequently found in college students than in peers who are not in college. Suicide is more frequently found in warm climates than colder ones, occurs more in the higher than in the lower socioeconomic classes, and is often related to the high expectations that can cause severe disappointment. Baumeister sees this disappointment or loss as an initial step in a long chain of events which lead to suicide: experiencing a loss and disappointment; attributing the cause of loss to oneself; mental narrowing; withdrawal; and finally suicide as an escape from an adverse situation and a damaged sense of self. Baumeister's thoughtful theory is worth consideration.

There are some risk factors that therapists are well advised to keep in mind. If a patient has made a suicidal attempt or gesture, discussed a threatened suicide, described a plan to take his or her life, or is preoccupied with death, the therapist should be attentive to suicidal risk. Other factors to watch for are a patient's proximity to violence or suicide; alcohol and drug abuse; impulsive and antisocial behavior patterns; a recent severe stress, loss, or disappointment; hopelessness as perhaps reflected by a lack of future plans; access to instruments of death, such as a gun, car, or drugs, particularly in impulsive patients.

It should be recalled, however, that risk factors only increase the likelihood of such actions, and do not determine such outcomes. Rich, Young, Fowler, Wagner, and Black (1990) have shown that gun control does not seem to affect the prevalence rate for suicide. Suicidal men, who are more likely to use guns than suicidal women, tend to turn to jumping from high places when guns are not available.

Responses to Suicidal Risks

If suicide is assessed as a risk, it raises the question of what to do. It seems clear that intervening directly is indicated if the risk of suicide is severe, regardless of any possible harm to a therapeutic relationship. Maintaining physical safety must always be the highest priority in any treatment.

We recommend that the matter of suicide be discussed directly with the patient. Hints of suicidal thoughts should be confronted immediately, particularly with high-risk patients. Further, the higher the risk the more active the therapist should be and the more immediate the response should be. Assessing any plan for suicide and the possible instrumentality seems important. Some assessment of lethality of risk can be derived from this information. The greater the lethality, the more specific the plan, the easier the access to instrumentalities for suicide, then the more immediate, direct, and aggressive the intervention should be.

It should also be remembered that many of those with depression who are at risk for suicide have major depressive problems, and a high percentage of these patients are psychotic. Psychosis can wax and wane during the course of a syndrome. Any patients who are suicidal should also be reviewed and screened for psychosis, including the presence of hallucinations or delusions.

A decision must be made for inpatient or outpatient treatment. The informed provider who can effectively treat the suicidal and depressed patient needs to know the procedures for involuntary commitment. In some states, individuals must be referred to those designated to assess and exercise the power to hospitalize someone against his or her will. In other states, a wider variety of mental health professionals are authorized to perform commitment procedures. Having familiarity with not only the concept but the specifics of the involuntary commitment process is important. Not merely knowing that a specific person should be contacted if a patient is suicidal, but knowing how to contact that person, where the phone number is, and the likely length of time before a response are specific bits of information that may be vital.

In a managed care context one also needs to know about details of access to approved inpatient treatment. Though certainly not of the utmost immediate relevance when a patient is suicidal, a hospitalization costing tens of thousands of dollars that could have been covered by an insurance company had the treating provider only known the procedures to use, could become quite important to a patient less depressed, more assertive, and in closer contact with legal resources.

Safety needs to be maintained. We find that reducing the presence of cues and instrumentalities is important. It is often helpful to get the family or life partners involved in this. Any increase in supportive social contact is helpful in reducing immediate suicidal risk in the short term. Getting a friend or family members to stay with the patient can help. Staying in touch with the patient through phone calls or direct follow-up is important. Having a backup plan for times when the therapist is not avilable is also important.

A contract not to attempt suicide can be very useful. Some find it helpful to write these contracts out in the presence of patients. Other practitioners are quite comfortable with a handshake and a personal direct gaze, but the commitment should be clear. Particularly with the patient with a dual diagnosis who may be somewhat manipulative in his or her approach to relationships, the promise to "call before I attempt suicide" may result merely in the passively aggressive patient leaving a message with one's answering service and then completing suicide. (The authors have heard of a faxed suicide note.) Get a commitment, a real one, even if only for a few days, that your patient will not attempt suicide.

It is sometimes possible to intervene therapeutically. Linehan (1993) looks at different dynamics between what she refers to as suicidal acts that are more "respondent" and those that are more "operant." Using a behavioral paradigm, she refers to respondent suicides as those in which there is a reaction to an external event. A person may react to something, experience the mental narrowing and numbing described by Baumeister, and the suicidal behavior is, if completed, a function of the prior environmental situation. The patient would be responding to environmental events.

An operant suicidal act is one in which the consequences of the behavior control the behavior. Here an individual might be seen as acting upon rather than merely reacting to the environment. The "respondent" suicidal patient may be characterized as more "wounded," and the "operant" suicidal patient may be characterized as somewhat more manipulative. One can hypothesize that parasuicidal behaviors may be more operant, in that they have a symbolic effect upon others. The patient's view of the social consequences of an attempted suicide or an announced plan may need to be addressed.

Adler (1956), for example, notes the importance of revenge as a motive in suicide and believes that people often commit suicide *at* another person. Adler finds it helpful to dispute the future social consequences of suicide that a patient may imagine, noting that the survivors may not be as wounded or as hurt as the patient believes, but may go on with their lives in his or her absence. It is possible to reframe or reconstrue a patient's motivation so that suicide is less acceptable to them. For example, with the patient who is attempting to portray such an act as a noble one, insisting that they don't wish to be a bother to anyone any longer, a redefinition of the suicide as a hostile act directed towards others regarded as unsupportive may lessen the suicidal motivation. This approach may not be effective, however, with the patient who is more withdrawn and cognitively inefficient. With one who is attempting to escape from life, rather than have an effect on it, such as a person with severe and chronic pain, such interventions may be counterproductive. Assessment of the dynamics of the suicidal patient is vital.

It makes sense to tell people not to commit suicide. One must be clear about this and insist that suicide is a bad idea. The therapist must be unwavering in this position, since some who deal with suicide (Quinnett, 1987) are quite clear that some suicidal patients are looking for permission to kill themselves and collusion from a therapist may provide it.

It is particularly important with suicidal patients to be attentive to respectful interactions. Suicidal patients are particularly attentive to rejection and may use signs of rejection, particularly from the therapist, as justification to finalize their plans. Disrespect can also be shown by failing to return phone calls, running late for appointments without explanation or apology, appearing bored, or any of a number of actions that may severely affect a patient's sense of acceptance, mutuality, and respect. Suicidal patients are often depressed, and depressed patients are seldom fun. The counterreactions of the therapist are particularly important. One should be attentive to the anger and manipulativeness of these patients. It is easy to get irked at them. Their behavior must be understood to be a part of the disease, and the therapist must remember to seek expert advice should these reactions become more intense.

Patients often need a sense of greater control over social situations. Some even see suicide as an attempt to overcome helplessness, controlling that which they always can control, their own mortality. Reframing or reconstructing the precipitating event as one that they can ultimately control, or as one which has a different meaning, may be helpful. Reducing one's sense of helplessness instills hope.

Since hopelessness is a component to suicide, encouraging hope and realistic optimism is important. Explaining that depression is an illness that can be managed may help a patient realize that there will be more obvious alternatives later. Suicide is often seen as a solution, though a bad one. Noted suicidologist Paul Quinnett (1987) observes that suicide is an attempt to solve a problem, and treatment with such patients necessitates coming up with a better solution. As he says, suicidal thoughts and plans may mean that something needs to die, but it shouldn't be the patient. It may be a job, a relationship, a view of oneself, a goal, or a plan, but not the patient.

Conclusion

Managed care is manageable. The rules are different, the tools are different, but the goals are the same. The dedicated mental health professional, committed to enhancing a person's fulfillment, satisfaction, and effectiveness, can still play a role in the managed care treatment context. Patients can gain benefit, and practitioners can gain reimbursement for their helpful efforts. Many things will be different, however, and flexibility may be the key to survival.

This is generally seen as a bleak time for mental health professionals, but it need not be so. As with any situation, change brings chaos, concerns, and stress, as well as the possibility for growth and betterment. One can even see the imposition of managed care as something akin to a Rorschach test. With the inkblot it is an interaction of the stimulus and the observer that produces the response. The same is true of managed care. There is real opportunity here for the creative, effective, and prepared provider. There is little opportunity, however, for the providers who insist upon merely doing it their way rather than to focus on the realistic needs of the patient, the community, and the purchasers of health care, who have collectively argued for and created a different treatment world.

In the past many therapists could attempt to help patients by providing a less task-focused but highly supportive relationship. Reimbursement for such a "process approach" to therapy will be harder and harder to find. Purchasers of health care will be shopping for outcomes, not procedures. They will purchase the most efficient programs that can document significant benefits to patients.

This is a world that will draw heavily upon knowledge. Knowledge of syndromes and interventions will be essential in an increasingly specialized world of focused care. As expertise becomes the requirement, more specialized and limited domains of expertise will likely be encouraged. It has been said that the heavens used to be occupied by angels, but now they are occupied by experts. So, too, might managed mental health care be increasingly occupied by specialists rather than friends.

Although this is also a world of specialization, those who think in terms of systems and appreciate part–whole relationships will do best in it. The expert who integrates such specialized knowledge into the real world context of a complex human being is the one who will effectively produce desired outcomes. The best academic psychopharmacologist will need to know something about medicine adherence and risk of misuse and have the capacity to develop an alliance with the patient who must actually fill the prescription and take the medicines conscientiously. The therapist who provides an intervention without documentation will have completed, in effect, an administratively invisible action, one which will be unlikely to receive reimbursement. The therapist who is unaware of other resources in the community or treatment team will be ineffectual, much as if a mechanic were limited to only one tool with which to complete a complicated repair.

Flexibility is essential. It is the palm tree that survives the hurricane, not the rigid oak. These are times of high winds, requiring the capacity to adapt. Those familiar with intrapsychic or psychosocial interventions will have to come to terms with the reality that medicines have a proven effect on certain populations of patients with depressive disorders. The biologically oriented physician will need to acknowledge the psychosocial aspects of patient care and treatment and admit that some therapeutic responses may be more effective than are others in certain circumstances.

Hierarchy will need to be dealt with in a different way than has been the tradition in health care. This is team treatment. Managed care will involve many practitioners with different levels of training, each contributing to the collective approach to patient needs which will be demanded in a sophisticated delivery system. Dogma and rank will be less adaptive in such a system than are attitudes of cooperation among peers and stature based on the therapeutic task of the moment.

There is probably something good to all this in terms of helping encourage a dedication to outcome, but the very human quality of mental health work cannot be lost. It is not enough to be merely knowledgeable. Both brightness and kindness will matter. As has been said, people die of cold, not of darkness. It is incumbent upon the therapist to bring this warmth, concern, respect, and regard to the therapeutic relationship, since only people, and not institutions, have a heart.

References

Abou-Saleh, M., & Coppen, A. (1983). Classification of depression and response to antidepressant therapies. *British Journal of Psychiatry, 143,* 601–603.

Abraham, K. (1911/1985). Notes on the psychoanalytic investigation and treatment of manic-depressive insanity and allied conditions. In J. C. Coyne (Ed.), *Essential papers on depression* (pp. 31–48). New York: New York University Press.

Abramson, L. Y, Alloy, L. B., & Metalsky, G. I. (1988). The cognitive diathesis stress theories of depression: Toward an adequate evaluation of the theories' validities. In L. B. Alloy (Ed.), *Cognitive processes in depression* (pp. 3–30). New York: Guilford Press.

Abramson, L. Y., Metalsky, G. I., & Alloy, L. B. (1993). Hopelessness. In C. G. Costello (Ed.), *Symptoms of depression* (pp. 181–205). New York: Wiley.

Abramson, L. Y., Seligman, M. E. P., & Teasdale, J. (1978). Learned helplessness in humans: Critique and reformulation. *Journal of Abnormal Psychology, 87,* 49–74.

Abramson, L. Y., Seligman, M. E. P., & Teasdale, J. D. (1986). Learned helplessness in humans: Critique and reformulation. In J. C. Coyne (Ed.), *Essential papers on depression* (pp. 259–301). New York: New York University Press.

Achenbach, T. M., & Edelbrock, C. S. (1983). *Manual for the child behavior checklist and the revised child behavior profile.* Burlington, VT: University Associates in Psychiatry.

Ackley, D. C. (1993). Managed care and outpatient mental health: The hidden costs. *The Independent Practioner, 13*(4), 155–159.

Adler, A. (1956). *The individual psychology of Alfred Adler.* (H. L. Ansbacher & R. R. Ansbacher, Eds.). New York: Basic Books.

Adler, A. (1964). *Social interest.* New York: Capricorn Books.

Adler, A. (1978). *Cooperation between the sexes.* (H. L. Ansbacher & R. R. Ansbacher, Eds.). Garden City, NY: Anchor.

189

Adler, G., & Gattaz, W. (1993). Pain perception threshold in major depression. *Biological Psychiatry, 34*(10), 687–689.

Akiskal, H. (1985). A proposed clinical approach to chronic and "resistant" depressions: Evaluation and treatment. *Journal of Clinical Psychiatry, 46,* 32–36.

Alberti, R. E., & Emmons, M. (1974). *Your perfect right* (2nd ed.). San Luis Obispo, CA: Impact.

Alexopoulos, G. S. (1994). Psychobiology of affective disorders. In V. D. Volkan (Ed.), *Depressive states and their treatment* (pp. 337–358). Northvale, NJ: Jason Aronson.

Allen, A., & Skinner, H. (1987). Lifestyle assessments using microcomputers. In J. Butcher (Ed.), *Computerized psychological assessment* (pp. 117–132). New York: Basic Books.

Altamura, A., & Mauri, M. (1985). Plasma concentrations, information and therapy adherence during long-term treatment with antidepressants. *British Journal of Clinical Pharmacology, 20*(6), 714–716.

Alvine, R. (1989). Data watch: Labor issues for the 1990s. *Business & Health, 7,* 12.

American Psychiatric Association. (1980). *Diagnostic and statistical manual of mental disorders* (3rd ed.). Washington, DC: Author.

American Psychiatric Association. (1987). *Diagnostic and statistical manual of mental disorders* (3rd ed. rev.). Washington, DC: Author.

American Psychiatric Association. (1990). *APA Task Force report on the practice of electroconvulsive therapy.* Washington, DC: Author.

American Psychiatric Association. (1994). *Diagnostic and statistical manual of mental disorders* (4th ed.). Washington, DC: Author.

American Psychological Association. (1994). *APA member focus groups on the health care environment: A summary report.* Washington, DC: Widmeyer Group.

Amsterdam, J., Brunswick, D., & Mendels, J. (1980). The clinical application of tricyclic antidepressant pharmacokinetics and plasma levels. *American Journal of Psychiatry, 137,* 653–662.

Anderson, J. C., Williams, S., McGee, R., & Silva, P. A. (1987). DSM-III disorders in preadolescent children: Prevalence in a large sample from the general population. *Archives of General Psychiatry, 44,* 69–76.

Aneshensel, C. S., Frerichs, R. R., & Clark, V. A. (1981). Family roles and sex differences in depression. *Journal of Health and Social Behavior, 22*(4), 379–393.

Angst, J., & Dobler-Mikola, A. (1985). The Zurich study: VI. A continuum from depression to anxiety disorders? *European Archives of Psychiatry & Clinical Neuroscience, 235*(3), 179–186.

Anthony, D. (1992). A retrospective evaluation of factors influencing successful outcomes on an inpatient psychiatric crisis unit. *Research on Social Work Practice, 2*(1), 56–64.

Ardid, D., Marty, H., Fialip, J., Privat, A. M., Eschalier, A., & Lavarenne, J. (1992). Comparative effects of different uptake inhibitor antidepressants in two pain tests in mice. *Fundamental and Clinical Pharmacology, 6*(2), 75–82.

Arieti, S., & Bemporad, J. (1978). *Severe and mild depression: The psychotherapeutic approach.* New York: Basic Books.

Asberg, M., & Bertilsson, L. (1979). Serotonin in depressive illness: Studies of CSF 5-HIAA. In B. Saleto, P. Berner, & L. E. Hollister (Eds.), *Neuropsychopharmacology* (pp. 105–115). New York: Pergamon Press.

Asher, S. J., Huffaker, G. Q., & McNally, M. (1994). Therapeutic considerations of wilderness therapy for women: The power of adventure. *Women & Therapy, 15*(3–4), 161–174.

Austad, C. S., & Hoyt, M. F. (1992). The managed care movement and the future of psychotherapy. *Psychotherapy, 29*(1), 109.

Ballenger, J. (1994). *Panic disorder, social phobia and depression: The clinical interface.* Mississauga, Ontario: Canadian Psychiatric Association, 17–23.

Bandura A. (1977). *Social learning theory.* Englewood Cliffs, NJ: Prentice-Hall.

Bant, W. (1978). Antihypertensive drugs and depression: A reappraisal. *Psychological Medicine, 8,* 275–283.

Barbee, J. (1994). Memory impairment and benzodiazephines. *Audio-Digest, Psychiatry, 23*(02).

Barklage, N. E. (1993). The new mood stabilizers have blemishes: Side effects and drug interactions. *Audio-Digest, Psychiatry,* 22 (13).

Barlow, D. (1991). *The treatment of anxiety and panic disorders.* Conference sponsored by the Mid-Atlantic Educational Institute, Alsecon, NJ.

Barlow, J., Macy, S., & Struthers, G. (1993). Health locus of control, self-help and treatment adherence in relation to ankylosing spondylitis patients. *Patient Education & Counseling, 20*(2–3), 153–166.

Barrett, J. E., Barrett, J. A., Oxman, T., & Gerber, P. (1988). The prevalence of psychiatric disorders in a primary care practice. *Archives of General Psychiatry, 45,* 1100–1106.

Barrett, M. L., Berney, T. P., Bhate, S., Famuyiwa, O., Fundudis, T., Kolvin, I., & Tyrer, S. (1991). Diagnosing childhood depression: Who should be interviewed—parent or child? The Newcastle Child Depression Project. *British Journal of Psychiatry, 159* (Suppl. 11), 22–27.

Bateson, G. (1972). *Steps to an ecology of mind.* New York: Ballantine.

Baumeister, R. F. (1993). Suicide attempts. In C. G. Costello (Ed.), *Symptoms of depression* (pp. 259–289). New York: Wiley.

Baxter, L. R. Jr., Schwartz, J. M., Guze, B. H., Bergman, K., & Szuba, M. P. (1990). PET imaging in patients with compulsive disorder with and without depression. *Journal of Clinical Psychiatry, 51*(Suppl.), 61.

Baxter, L. R. Jr., Schwartz, J. M., Phelps, M. E., Mazziotta, J. C., Guze, B. H., Selin, C. E., Gerner, R. H., & Sumida, R. M. (1989). Reduction of prefrontal cortex glucose metabolism common to three types of depression. *Archives of General Psychiatry, 46,* 243–250.

Beach, S., Arias, I., & O'Leary, K. (1983). *Risk for depression as a factor of social support.* Paper presented at the meeting of the Eastern Psychological Association, Philadelphia.

Beardsley, R. S., Gardocki, G. J., Larson, D. B., & Hidalgo, J. (1988). Prescribing of psychotropic medication by primary care physicians and psychiatrists. *Archives of General Psychiatry, 45*(12), 1117–1119.

Beasley, C., Sayler, M., Cunningham, G., Weiss, A., & Masica, D. (1990).

Fluoxetine in tricyclic refractory major depressive disorder. *Journal of Affective Disorders, 20,* 193–200.

Bech, P., Kastrup, M., & Rafaelsen, O. J. (1986). Mini-compendium of rating scales for anxiety, depression, mania, schizophrenia with corresponding DSM-III syndromes. *Acta Psychiatrica Scandinavica, 73,* 1–39.

Beck, A. T. (1964). Thinking and depression: 2. Theory and therapy. *Archives of General Psychiatry, 10,* 561–571.

Beck, A. T. (1967). *Depression: Clinical, experimental, and theoretical aspects.* New York: Harper & Row.

Beck, A. T. (1976). *Cognitive therapy and the emotional disorders.* New York: International Universities Press.

Beck, A. T., Hollon, S. D., Young, J. E., Bedrosian, R. C., & Budenz, D. (1985). Treatment of depression with cognitive therapy and amitriptyline. *Archives of General Psychiatry, 42,* 142–148.

Beck, A. T., Rush, A. J., Shaw, B. F., & Emery, G. (1979). *Cognitive therapy of depression.* New York: Guilford Press.

Beck, A. T., Steer, R. A., & Garbin, M. G. (1988). Psychometric properties of the Beck Depression Inventory: 25 years of evaluation. *Clinical Psychology Review, 8,* 77–100.

Beck, A. T., Ward, C. H., Mendelson, M., Mock, J., & Erbaugh, J. (1961). An inventory for measuring depression. *Archives of General Psychiatry, 4,* 561–571.

Becker, E. S. (1986). Depression: A comprehensive theory. In J. C. Coyne (Ed.), *Essential papers on depression* (pp. 366–389). New York: New York University Press.

Becker, J., & Kleinman, A. (1991). *Psychosocial aspects of depression.* Hillsdale, NJ: Erlbaum.

Beckham, E., & Leber, W. (1985). *Handbook of depression: Treatment, assessment, and research.* Homewood, IL: Dorsey Press.

Belar, C. (1991). Behavioral medicine. In W. Berman & C. Austad (Eds.), *Psychotherapy in managed health care: The optimal use of time and resources.* Washington, DC: American Psychological Association Press.

Bellack, A., Hersen, M., & Himmelhoch, J. (1983). A comparison of social-skills training, pharmacotherapy and psychotherapy for depression. *Behavior Research & Therapy, 21*(2), 101–107.

Benbow, S. M. (1987). The use of electroconvulsive therapy in old age psychiatry. *International Journal of Geriatric Psychiatry, 2,* 25–30.

Berg-Cross, L., Jennings, P., & Baruch, R. (1990). Cinematherapy: Theory and application. Presented at the 96th annual meeting of the American Psychological Association, Psychotherapy supervisions: Professional and ethical issues (1988, Atlanta, GA). *Psychotherapy in Private Practice, 8*(1), 135–156.

Bergin, A. E. (1980). Negative effects revisited: A reply. *Professional Psychology, 11*(1), 93–100.

Berman, K. (1987). Health insurance rates keep climbing. *Business Insurance, 21,* 1, 34.

Bernadt, M. W., & Murray, R. M. (1986). Psychiatric disorder, drinking and alcoholism: What are the links? *British Journal of Psychiatry, 148,* 393–400.

Berndt, D. J. (1986). *Multiscore Depression Inventory manual.* Los Angeles: Western Psychological Services.

Berndt, D. J. (1990). Inventories and scales. In B. B. Wolman & G. Stricker (Eds.), *Depressive disorders: Facts, theories, and treatment methods* (pp. 255–274). New York: Wiley.

Berndt, S., Maier, C., & Schutz, H. (1993). Polymedication and medication compliance in patients with chronic non-malignant pain. *Pain, 52*(3), 311–339.

Bernet, C. Z., Ingram, R. E., & Johnson, B. R. (1993). Self-esteem. In C. G. Costello (Ed.), *Symptoms of depression* (pp. 141–159). New York: Wiley.

Bernstein, G. A. (1991). Comorbidity and severity of anxiety and depressive disorders in a clinic population. *Journal of the American Academy of Child Psychiatry, 30,* 43–50.

Beskow, J., Gottfries, C. G., Roos, B. E., & Winblad, D. B. (1976). Determination of monoamine and monamine metabolites in the human brain: Post-mortem studies in a group of suicides and in a control group. *Acta Psychiatrica Scandinavia, 53,* 7–20.

Biegel, D. E., et al. (1995). A comparative analysis of family caregivers' perceived relationships with mental health professionals. *Psychiatric Services, 46,* 477–482.

Bielski, R., Major, J., & Rice, J. (1992). Phototherapy with broad spectrum white florescent light: A comparative study. *Psychiatry Research, 43*(2), 167–175.

Bifulco, A. T., Brown, G. W., & Harris, T. (1987). Childhood loss of parent, lack of adequate parental care and adult depression: A replication. *Journal of Affective Disorders, 12,* 115–128.

Billings, A. G., Cronkite, R., & Moos, R. (1983). Social–environmental factors in unipolar depression: Comparisons of depressed patients and nondepressed controls. *Journal of Abnormal Psychology, 93,* 119–133.

Billings, A. G., & Moos, R. H. (1985). Psychosocial processes of remission in unipolar depression: Comparing depressed patients with matched community controls. *Journal of Consulting and Clinical Psychology, 53,* 314–325.

Billings, A. G., & Moos, R. H. (1986). Psychosocial theory and research on depression: An integrative framework and review. In J. C. Coyne (Ed.), *Essential papers on depression* (pp. 331–365). New York: New York University Press.

Billings, A. G., Moos, R., Cronkite, R., & Waring, E. (1994). The role of marital therapy in the treatment of depressed married women. *Canadian Journal of Psychiatry, 39*(9), 568–576.

Black, D., Bell, S., Hulbert, J., & Nasrallah, A. (1988). The importance of Axis II in patients with major depression: A controlled study. *Journal of Affective Disorders, 14*(2), 115–122.

Blackburn, I., Bishop, S., Glen, A., Whalley, L., & Christie, J. (1981). The efficacy of cognitive therapy in depression: A treatment trial using cognitive therapy and pharmacotherapy, each alone and in combination. *British Journal of Psychiatry, 139,* 181–189.

Blackburn, I., Eunson, K., & Bishop, S. (1986). A two-year naturalistic follow-up of depressed patients treated with cognitive therapy, pharmacotherapy and a combination of both. *Journal of Affective Disorders, 10,* 67–75.

Blacker, C., & Clare, A. (1988). The prevalence and treatment of depression in general practice. *Psychopharmacology, 95,* 514–517.

Blazer, D. (1993). *Depression in later life.* St. Louis, MO: Mosby-YearBook.

Blazer, D. G., Bachar, J. R., & Manton, K. G. (1986). Suicide in late life: Review and commentary. *Journal of the American Geriatric Society, 34,* 519–525.

Blazer, D., Hughes, D. C., & George, L. K. (1987). The epidemiology of depression in an elderly community population. *Gerontologist, 27,* 281–287.

Blumberg, S. R., & Hokanson, J. E. (1983). The effects of another person's response style on interpersonal behavior in depression. *Journal of Abnormal Psychology, 92,* 196–209.

Blumenthal, J., Williams, R., Wallace, A., Williams, R., Jr., & Needles, T. (1982). Physiological and psychological variables predict compliance to prescribed exercise therapy in patients recovering from myocardial infarction. *Psychosomatic Medicine, 44*(6), 519–527.

Borkovec, T. D., & Boudewyns, P. A. (1976). Treatment of insomnia with stimulus control and progressive relaxation procedures. In J. D. Krumbolz & C. Thoresen (Eds.), *Counseling methods* (pp. 103–126). New York: Holt, Reinhart and Winston.

Bornstein, P. H., & Bornstein, M. T. (1986). *Marital therapy: A behavioral communications approach.* New York: Pergamon Press.

Borus, J. F., & Olendzki, M. C. (1985). The offset effect of mental health treatment on ambulatory medical care utilization and charges. *Archives of General Psychiatry, 42,* 573–580.

Bosscher, R. J. (1993). Running and mixed physical exercises with depressed psychiatric patients. *International Journal of Sport Psychology, 24*(2), 170–184.

Boswell, P. C., & Murray, E. J. (1981). Depression, schizophrenia, and social attraction. *Journal of Consulting and Clinical Psychology, 49,* 641–647.

Bothwell, S., & Weissman, M. (1977). Social impairments four years after an acute depressive episode. *American Journal of Orthopsychiatry, 47,* 231–237.

Bourin, M., Kergueris, M., & Lapierre, Y. (1989). Therapeutic monitoring of treatment with antidepressants. *Psychiatric Journal of the University of Ottawa, 14,* 460–462.

Bourne, H. R., Bunney, W. E., & Colburn, R. W. (1968). 5–hydroxytryptamine and 5–hydroxindoleacetic acid in the hind brains of suicidal patients. *Lancet, 2,* 805–808.

Bowen, M. (1981). Theory in the practice of psychotherapy. In G. Berenson & H. White (Eds.), *Annual review of family therapy, Vol. 1* (pp. 82–103). New York: Human Sciences Press.

Bower, G. H. (1981). Mood and memory. *American Psychologist, 36,* 129–148.

Boyer, W. (1994). Managing depression in 1994. *Audio-Digest, Internal Medicine, 41*(01).

Boza, R., Milanes, F., Hanna, S., Kaye, J., & Jonas, E. A. (1989). Noncompliance in chronic depression: Assessment of serum antidepressant determination with the enzyme-immunoassay method. Presented at the meeting of the American Academy of Clinical Psychiatrists (1988, Seattle, WA). *Annals of Clinical Psychiatry, 1*(1), 43–49.

Breier, A., Kelsoe, J. R., Jr., Kirwin, P. D., Beller, S. A., Wolkowitz, O. M., & Pickar, D. (1988). Early parental loss and development of adult psychopathology. *Archives of General Psychiatry, 45,* 987–993.

Brewin, C. R. (1985). Depression and casual attributions: What is their relation? *Psychological Bulletin, 98,* 297–309.

Brewin, C. R. (1989). Cognitive change processes in psychotherapy. *Psychological Review, 96,* 379–394.

Bridges, K., & Goldberg, D. (1985). Somatic presentation of DSM-III psychiatric disorders in primary care. *Journal of Psychosomatic Research, 29*(6), 563–569.

Broadhead, W., Blazer, D., George, D., & Tse, C. (1990). Depression, disability days, and days lost from work in a prospective epidemiologic survey. *Journal of the American Medical Association, 246*(19), 2524–2528.

Broskowski, A. T. (1995). The evolution of health care: Implications for the training and careers of psychologists. *Professional Psychology: Research and Practice, 26,* 156–162.

Broughton, R. J. (1992). Psychosocial impact of narcolepsy-catalepsy with comparisons to idiopathic hypersomnia and epilepsy. *Loss, Grief, and Care, 5*(3–4), 37–43.

Brown, F. (1961). Depression and childhood bereavement. *Journal of Mental Science, 107,* 754–777.

Brown, G. W. (1986). A three-factor casual model of depression. In J. C. Coyne (Ed.), *Essential papers on depression* (pp. 390–402). New York: New York University Press.

Brown, G. W. (1991). Epidemiological studies of depression: Definition and case finding. In J. Becker & A. Kleinman (Eds.), *Psychosocial aspects of depression* (pp. 1–37). Hillsdale, NJ: Erlbaum.

Brown, G. W., Bifulco, A., & Harris, T. (1987). Life events, vulnerability and onset of depression: Some refinements. *British Journal of Psychiatry, 150,* 30–42.

Brown, G. W., & Harris, T. (1978). *Social origins of depression.* London: Free Press.

Brown, L. S., & Liss-Levinson, N. (1981). Feminist therapy I. In R. Corsini (Ed.), *Handbook of innovative psychotherapies* (pp. 299–314). New York: Wiley.

Brown, S. A., & Schuckit, M. A. (1988). Changes in depression among abstinent alcoholics. *Journal of Studies on Alcohol, 49*(5), 412–417.

Brown, W. A. (1990). Is light treatment a placebo? *Psychopharmacology Bulletin, 26,* 527.

Brugha, T. S., & Bebbington, P. E. (1992). The undertreatment of depression. *European Archives of Psychiatry and Clinical Neuroscience, 242*(2–3), 103–108.

Brugha, T. S., Conroy, R., Walsh, N., Delaney, W., O'Hanlon, J., Dondero, E., Daly, L., Hickey, N., & Bourke, G. (1982). Social networks, attachments and support in minor affective disorders: A replication. *British Journal of Psychiatry, 141,* 249–255.

Buchanan, A. (1992). A two-year prospective study of treatment compliance in patients with schizophrenia. *Psychological Medicine, 22*(3), 787–797.

Budman, S. H. (1981). *Forms of brief therapy.* New York: Guilford Press.

Budman, S. H., & Gurman, A. S. (1988). *Theory and practice of brief therapy.* New York: Guilford Press.

Burns, D., & Auerbach, A. (1992). Does homework compliance enhance recovery from depression? *Psychiatric Annals, 22*(9), 464–469.

Burns, D. D. (1980). *Feeling good: The new mood therapy.* New York: Avon Books.

Burns, M. O., & Seligman, M. E. P. (1989). Explanatory style across the lifespan: Evidence of stability over 52 years. *Journal of Personality and Social Psychology, 56,* 471–477.

Burton, W., Hoy, D., Bonin, R., & Gladstone, L. (1989). Quality and cost-effective management of mental health care. *Journal of Occupational Medicine, 31,* 363–366.

Butcher, J. N., & Koss, M. P. (1978). Research on brief and crisis-oriented therapies. In S. Garfield & A. E. Bergin (Eds.), *Handbook of psychotherapy and behavior change* (2nd ed., pp. 725–768). New York: Wiley.

Byrne, A., & Byrne, D. (1993). The effect of exercise on depression, anxiety and other mood states: A review. *Journal of Psychosomatic Research, 37*(6), 565–574.

Cade, B., & O'Hanlon, W. H. (1993). *A brief guide to brief therapy.* New York: Norton.

Cadoret, R. (1978). Evidence of genetic inheritance of primary affective disorder in adoptees. *American Journal of Psychiatry, 135,* 463–466.

Caillard, V. (1990). Syndromes depressifs et antidepresseurs. [Depressive syndromes and antidepressants]. *European Psychiatry, 5*(6), 355–362.

Campbell, S. S., Terman, M., Lewy, A. J., Kijk, D. J., Eastman, C. I., & Boulos, Z. (1995). Light treatment for sleep disorders: Consensus report. V. Age-related disturbances. *Journal of Biological Rhythms, 10*(2), 151–154.

Campbell, T. W. (1992). Therapeutic relationships and iatrogenic outcomes: The blame-and-change maneuver in psychotherapy. *Psychotherapy, 29*(3), 474–480.

Cantor, P. C. (1972). *Personality and status characteristics of the female youthful suicide attempter.* Unpublished doctoral dissertation, Columbia University, New York.

Cantor, P. C. (1990). Symptoms, prevention, and treatment of attempted suicide. In B. B. Wolman & G. Stricker (Eds.), *Depressive disorders: Facts, theories, and treatment methods* (pp. 189–202). New York: Wiley.

Cantwell, D. P. (1994). Depression in adolescents/comorbidity in mania. *Audio-Digest, Psychiatry 23* (9).

Carlson, G. A. (1990). Child and adolescent mania–diagnostic considerations. *Journal of Child Psychology and Psychiatry, 31,* 331–341.

Carlson, G. A., & Cantwell, D. P. (1980). A survey of depressive symptoms, syndrome and disorder in a child psychiatric population. *Journal of Child Psychology and Psychiatry, 21,* 19–25.

Carlson, G. A., & Garber, J. (1986). Developmental issues in the classification of depression in children. In M. Rutter, C. E. Izard, & P. B. Read (Eds.), *Depression in young people: Developmental and clinical perspectives* (pp. 399–434). New York: Guilford Press.

Carlson, G. A., & Kashani, J. H. (1988). Phenomenology of major depression from childhood through adulthood: Analysis of three studies. *American Journal of Psychiatry, 145,* 1222–1225.

Carr, J. E. (1995, May 5). Anxiety vs. panic: The same or different syndromes?

Talk given at the Mental Health Update, *Psyche or soma? Difficult differential diagnoses*. University of Washington, Seattle.

Carr, V., Dorrington, C., Schader, G., & Wale, J. (1983). The use of ECT in childhood bipolar disorder. *British Journal of Psychiatry, 143*, 411–415.

Carroll, B. J., Fielding, J. M., & Blashki, T. G. (1973). Depression rating scales: A critical review. *Archives of General Psychiatry, 28*, 361–366.

Cartwright, R. D. (1993). Sleeping problems. In C. G. Costello (Ed.), *Symptoms of depression* (pp. 243–257). New York: Wiley.

Casey, D. A. (1993). Diagnosis of depression in the elderly. *Audio-Digest, Psychiatry, 22* (17).

Castellano, T. C., & Soderstrom, I. R. (1992). Therapeutic wilderness programs and juvenile recidivism: A program evaluation. *Journal of Offender Rehabilitation, 17*(3–4), 19–46.

Clark, L. A., & Watson, D. (1991). Theoretical and empirical issues in differentiating depression from anxiety. In J. Becker & A. Kleinman (Eds.), *Psychosocial aspects of depression* (pp. 39–65). Hillsdale, NJ: Erlbaum.

Claussen, J., & Yarrow, M. (1955). Introduction: Mental illness and the family. *Journal of Social Issues, 11*, 3–5.

Cloitre, M., Katz, M. M., & Van Praag, H. M. (1993). Psychomotor agitation and retardation. In C. G. Costello (Ed.), *Symptoms of depression* (pp. 207–226). New York: Wiley.

Coffey, B. J. (1995). Anxiolytics. *Audio-Digest, Psychiatry, 24* (07).

Cohler, B. J., & Boxer, A. M. (1984). Middle adulthood: Settling into the world—person, time, and context. In D. Offer & M. Sabshin (Eds.), *Normality and the life cycle* (pp. 145–203). New York: Basic Books.

Cohn, J., & Wilcox, C. (1985). A comparison of fluoxetine, imipramine, and placebo in patients with major depressive disorder. *Journal of Clinical Psychiatry, 46*(3, Part 2), 26–31.

Cole, J. O. (1970). Clinical uses of the amphetamines. In E. H. Ellinwood & S. Cohen (Eds.), *Current concepts on amphetimine abuse: Proceedings of a workshop at Duke University Medical Center, June 5–6, 1970*. Washington, DC: U.S. Government Printing Office.

Coll, P. G., & Bland, R. C. (1979). Manic depressive illness in adolescence and childhood: Review and case report. *Canadian Journal of Psychiatry, 24*(3), 255–263.

Conn, V., Taylor, S., & Kelley, S. (1991). Medication regimen complexity and adherence among older adults. *IMAGE: Journal of Nursing Scholarship, 23*(4), 231–235.

Copeland, M. E. (1994). *Living without depression and manic depression: A workbook for maintaining mood stability*. Oakland, CA: New Harbinger Publications.

Coppen, A., Abou-Saleh, M. T., Millin, P., Bailey, J., Metcalfe, M., Burns, B. H., & Armond, A. (1981). A lithium continuation therapy following electroconvulsive therapy. *British Journal of Psychiatry, 139*, 284–287.

Coppen, A., Mendelwicz, J., & Kielholz, P. (1986). *Pharmacotherapy of depressive disorders: A consensus statement.* Geneva, Switzerland: World Health Organization.

Corsini, R. J. (1981). *Handbook of innovative psychotherapies.* New York: Wiley.

Coryell, W. R., Noyes, R., & Cancy, J. (1982). Excess mortality in panic disorder: A comparison with primary unipolar depression. *Archives of General Psychiatry, 39,* 701–703.

Costello, C. G. (1972). Depression: Loss of reinforcers or loss of reinforcer effectiveness? *Behavior Therapy, 3,* 240–247.

Costello, C. G. (1993). *Symptoms of depression.* New York: Wiley.

Coulehan, J. L., Schulberg, H. C., & Block, M. R. (1989). The efficiency of depression questionnaires for case finding in primary medical care. *Journal of General Internal Medicine, 4,* 542–547.

Coulehan, J. L., Schulberg, H. C., Block, M. R., Janosky, J. E., & Arena, V. C. (1990). Medical comorbidity of major depressive disorder in a primary medical practice. *Archives of Internal Medicine, 150,* 2363–2367.

Covi, L., & Lipman, R. (1987). Cognitive behavioral group psychotherapy combined with imipramine in major depression. *Psychopharmacology Bulletin, 23*(1), 173–176.

Coyne, J. C. (1976). Depression and the response of others. *Journal of Abnormal Psychology, 85,* 186–193.

Coyne, J. C. (1986). Toward an interactional description of depression. *Essential papers on depression* (pp. 311–330). New York: New York University Press.

Coyne, J. C., Schwenk, T. L., & Fechner-Bates, S. (1995). Nondetection of depression by primary care physicians reconsidered. *General Hospital Psychiatry, 17,* 3–12.

Craighead, W. E. (1991). Cognitive factors and classification issues in adolescent depression. *Journal of Youth & Adolescence, 20*(2), 311–326.

Craighead, W. E., Curry, J. F., & Ilardi, S. S. (1995). Relationship of children's depression inventory factors to major depression among adolescents. *Psychological Assessment, 7*(2), 171–176.

Croake, J. (1987). Working with couples in groups. *Individual Psychology, 43*(2), 206–209.

Croake, J., & Olson, T. (1977). Family constellation and personality. *Journal of Individual Psychology, 33*(1), 9–18.

Cummings, N. A. (1986). The dismantling of our health system: Strategies for the survival of psychological practice. *American Psychologist, 41,* 426–431.

Cummings, N. A. (1988). Emergence of the mental health complex: Adaptive and maladapative responses. *Professional Psychology: Research and Practice, 19,* 308–315.

Cummings, N. A. (1991). Intermittent therapy throughout the life cycle. In C. S. Austad & W. H. Berman (Eds.), *Psychotherapy in managed health care.* Washington, DC: American Psychological Association Press.

Cummings, N. A. (1995a). Behavioral health after managed care: The next golden opportunity for professional psychology. *Register Report, 20*(3) & *21*(1), 1, 30.

Cummings, N. A. (1995b). Impact of managed care on employment and training: A primer for survival. *Professional Psychology: Research and Practice, 26*(1), 10–15.

Cummings, N. A., Dorken, H., Pallak, M. S., & Henke, R. J. (1990). *The impact of psychological intervention on healthcare utilization.* San Francisco: Biodyne Institute.

Curtiss, F. (1989). How managed care works. *Personnel Journal, 68*, 38–53.

Cutrona, C. E. (1984). Social support and stress in the transition to parenthood. *Journal of Abnormal Psychology, 93*, 378–390.

Cytryn, L., & McKnew, D. H. (1972). Proposed classification of childhood depression. *American Journal of Psychiatry, 129*, 149–155.

Dalkvist, J., Wahlin, T. B., Bartsch, E., & Forsbeck, M. (1995). Herpes simplex and mood: A prospective study. *Psychosomatic Medicine, 57*(2), 127–137.

Dallal, A., Fontaine, R., Ontiveros, A., & Elie, R. (1990). Lithium carbonate augmentation of desipramine in refractory depression. *Canadian Journal of Psychiatry, 35*(7), 608–611.

Dangel, R. F., & Polster, R. A. (1988). *Teaching child management skills.* New York: Pergamon Press.

DasGupta, K. (1994). Managing side effects and toxicity of antidepressant drugs. *Audio-Digest, Psychiatry, 23* (18).

Davanloo, H. (1980). A method of short-term dynamic psychotherapy. In H. Davanloo (Ed.), *Short-term dynamic psychotherapy* (pp. 43–71). New York: Jason Aronson.

Davies, N. E., & Felder, L. H. (1990). Applying brakes to the runaway American health care system: A proposed agenda. *Journal of the American Medical Association, 263*(1), 73–76.

DeAlarcon, R. (1964). Hypochondriasis and depression in the aged. *Gerontology Clinic, 6*, 266–277.

Dean, C., & Kendell, R. (1981). The symptomatology of postpartum illness. *British Journal of Psychiatry, 139*, 128–133.

DeBerry, S. (1987). Necessary factors in psychotherapy: A model for understanding iatrogenic disturbances. *Journal of Contemporary Psychotherapy, 17*(4), 235–249.

DeLeon, P. H., VandenBos, G. R., & Bulatao, E. Q. (1991). Managed mental health care: A history of the federal policy initiative. *Professional Psychology: Research and Practice, 22*, 15–25.

Deming, W. E. (1986). *Out of the crisis.* Cambridge, MA: Massachusetts Institute of Technology Center for Advanced Engineering Study (CAES).

Depression Guideline Panel. (1993). *Depression in primary care: Volume 1. Detection and diagnosis* (AHCPR Publication No. 93-0550). Rockville, MD: U.S. Department of Health and Human Services.

Depression Guideline Panel. (1993). *Depression in primary care: Detection, diagnosis, and treatment.* (Technical Report Number 5). (AHCPR Publication No. 93-0552). Rockville, MD: U.S. Department of Health and Human Services, Public Health Services.

Derogatis, L. R., Lipman, R. S., & Covi, L. (1973). The SCL-90: An outpatient psychiatric rating scale. *Psychopharmacology Bulletin, 9*, 13–28.

deShazer, S. (1985). *Keys to solution in brief therapy.* New York: Norton.

DeVane, C. L. (1994). Pharmacogenetics and drug metabolism of newer antidepressant agents. *Journal of Clinical Psychiatry, 55*(Suppl. 12), 38–43.

Deykin, E., Levy, J., & Wells, V. (1987). Adolescent depression, alcohol and drug abuse. *American Journal of Public Health, 77*(2), 178–182.

de Zwann, M. (1992). Exercise and antidepressant serum levels. *Biological Psychiatry, 32*(2), 210–211.

DiGiacomo, S. (1992). Metaphor as illness: Postmodern dilemmas in the representation of body, mind and disorder. *Medical Anthropology, 14*(1), 109–137.

DiMascio, A., Weissman, M. M., Prusoff, B. A., Neu, C., Zwilling, M., & Klerman, G. L. (1979). Differential symptom reduction by drugs and psychotherapy in acute depression. *Archives of General Psychiatry, 36*, 1450–1456.

Dishman, R. (1982). Compliance/adherence in health-related exercise. *Health Psychology, 1*(3), 237–267.

Dobson, K. (1985). An analysis of anxiety and depression scales. *Journal of Personality Assessment, 49*(5), 522–527.

Dohrenwend, B. P., Shrout, P. E., Link, B., Martin, J., & Skodol, A. (1986). Overview and initial results from a risk-factor study of depression and schizophrenia. In J. E. Barrett (Ed.), *Mental disorder in the community: Progress and challenges.* New York: Guilford Press.

Dornseif, B., Dunlop, S., Potvin, J., & Wernicke, J. (1989). Effect of dose escalation after low-dose fluoxetine therapy. *Psychopharmacology Bulletin, 25*(1), 71–79.

Dorus, W., Kennedy, J., Gibbons, R., & Ravi, S. (1987). Symptoms and diagnosis of depression in alcoholics. *Alcoholism: Clinical and Experimental Research, 11*(2), 150–154.

Draine, J., & Solomon, P. (1994). Explaining attitudes toward medication compliance among a seriously mentally ill population. *Journal of Nervous & Mental Disease, 182*(1), 50–54.

Drum, D. J. (1995). Changes in the mental health service delivery and finance systems and resulting implications for the National Register. *Register Report, 20*(3) & *21*(1), 4.

Dubovsky, S. L., & Thomas, M. (1995). Serotonergic mechanisms and current and future psychiatric practice. *Journal of Clinical Psychiatry, 56*(Suppl. 2), 38–48.

Duffy, J. F. (1994, April). Psychologist defends dispensing of Prozac. *Psychiatric Times,* 50.

Dunner, D. L. (1986). Recent genetic studies of bipolar and unipolar depression. In J. C. Coyne (Ed.), *Essential papers on depression* (pp. 449–458). New York: New York University Press.

Dunner, D. L., & Schmaling, K. B. (1994, June–July). Treatment of dysthymia: Fluoxetine versus cognitive therapy. Presented at the XIXth Collegium Internationale Neuro-Psychopharmacologicum Congress, Washington, DC. *Neuropsychopharmacology, 10, 35 (Part 2),* 234S.

Dworkin, S., von Korff, M., & LeResche, L. (1990). Multiple pains and psychiatric disturbance. *Archives of General Psychiatry, 47,* 239–244.

Eastman, C. (1976). Behavioural formulations of depression. *Psychological Review, 83,* 277–291.

Eaton, W., Holzer, C., III, von Korff, M., Anthony, J., Helzer, J., George, L., Burnam, M., Boyd, J., Kessler, L., & Locke, B. (1984). The design of the Epidemiologic Catchment Area surveys. *Archives of General Psychiatry, 41,* 942–948.

Eaton, W., Regier, D., Locke, B., & Taube, C. (1981). The Epidemiological Catchment Area Program of the National Institute of Mental Health. *Public Health Report, 96,* 319–325.

Eckert, P. A. (1994). Cost control through quality improvement: The new challenge for psychology. *Professional Psychology: Research and Practice, 25,* 1, 3–8.

Edelbrock, C., Costello, A. J., Dulcan, M. K., Conover, M. C., & Kalas, R. (1986). Parent–child agreement on child psychiatric symptoms assessed via structured interview. *Journal of Child Psychology and Psychiatry, 27,* 181–190.

Egbunike, I. G., & Chaffee, B. J. (1990). Antidepressants in the management of chronic pain syndromes. *Pharmacotherapy, 10*(4), 262–270.

Eisenberg, L. (1992). Treating depression and anxiety in primary care. *New England Journal of Medicine, 326,* 1080–1083.

Elixhauser, A., Eisen, S., & Romeis, J. (1990). The effects of monitoring and feedback on compliance. American Public Health Association Conference (1988, Boston, MA). *Medical Care, 28*(10), 882–893.

Elkin, I., Shea, T., Watkins, J., Imber, S., Sotsky, S., Collins, J., Glass, D., Pikonis, P., Leber W., Docherty, J., Fiester, S., & Parloff, M. (1989). National Institute of Mental Health Treatment of Depression Collaborative Research Program: General effectiveness of treatments. *Archives of General Psychiatry, 46,* 971–982.

Ellis, A. (1962). *Reason and emotion in psychotherapy.* New York: Lyle Stuart.

Ellis, A. (1993). *Clinical application of Rational-Emotive Therapy.* New York: Institute for Rational-Emotive Therapy.

Ellis, A., & Harper, R. A. (1975). *A new guide to rational living.* North Hollywood, CA: Wilshire Books.

Endicott, J., & Spitzer, R. (1978). A diagnostic interview: The schedule for affective disorders and schizophrenia. *Archives of General Psychiatry, 35,* 837–844.

Erickson, M. H., & Rossi, E. L. (1981). *Experiencing hypnosis.* New York: Irvington.

Evans, D. L. (1993). Depression and medical illness. *Audio-Digest, Psychiatry, 22* (14).

Ewert, A. (1988). Reduction of trait anxiety through participation in Outward Bound. *Leisure Sciences, 10*(2), 107–117.

Ewusi-Mensah, I., Saunders, J. B., Wodak, A. D., Murray, R. M., & Williams, R. (1983). Psychiatric morbidity in patients with alcoholic liver disease. *British Medical Journal Clinical Research Education, 287*(6403), 1417–1419.

Eysenck, H., & Eysenck, S. B. G. (1968). *Manual for the Eysenck personality inventory.* San Diego, CA: Educational and Industrial Testing Service.

Faravelli, C., Albanesi, G., & Poli, E. (1986). Assessment of depression: A comparison of rating scales. *Journal of Affective Disorders, 11*(3), 245–253.

Fava, M., Rappe, S. M., Pava, J. A., Nierenberg, A. A., Alpert, J. E., & Rosenbaum, J. F. (1995). Relapse in patients on long-term fluoxetine treatment: Response to increased fluoxetine dose. *Journal of Clinical Psychiatry, 56*(2), 52–55.

Fava, M., Rosenbaum, J. F., McGrath, P. J., Stewart, J. W., Amsterdam, J. D., & Quitkin, F. M. (1994). Lithium and tricyclic augmentation of fluoxetine treatment for resistant major depression: A double-blind, controlled study. *American Journal of Psychiatry, 151*(9), 1372–1374.

Fawcett, J., Scheftner, W., Clark, D., Hedeker, D., Gibbons, R., & Coryell, W. (1987). Clinical prospective study. *American Journal of Psychiatry, 144*, 35–40.

Feighner, J. P. (1994). Actions of antidepressants. *Audio-Digest, Family Practice, 23* (03).

Feldman, E., Mayou, R., Hawton, K., Ardern, M., & Smith, E. (1987). Psychiatric disorder in medical inpatients. *Quarterly Journal of Medicine, 63*, 405–412.

Feldman, L. A., & Gotlib, I. H. (1993). Social dysfunction. In C. G. Costello (Ed.), *Symptoms of depression* (pp. 85–112). New York: Wiley.

Feldstein, P., Wickizer, T., & Wheeler, J. (1988). Private cost containment: The effects of utilization review programs on health care use and expenditures. *New England Journal of Medicine, 318*, 1310–1314.

Fensterheim, H., & Baer, J. (1975). *Don't say yes when you want to say no.* New York: Dell.

Ferster, C. B. (1966). Animal behaviour and mental illness. *Psychological Record, 16*, 345–356.

Fiedler, J. L., & Wight, J. B. (1989). *The medical offset effect and public health policy: Mental health industry in transition.* New York: Praeger.

Fiester, A. R., & Rudestam, K. E. (1975). A multivariate analysis of the early dropout process. *Journal of Consulting and Clinical Psychology, 43*, 528–535.

Fine, S., Forth, A., Gilbert, M., & Haley, G. (1991). Group therapy for adolescent depressive disorder: A comparison of social skills and therapeutic support. *Journal of the American Academy of Child Psychiatry, 30*, 79–85.

Fingeret, M., & Schuettenberg, S. (1991). Patient drug schedules and compliance. *Journal of the American Optometric Association, 62*(6), 478–480.

Finnegan, D., & Suler, J. (1985). Psychological factors associated with maintenance of improved health behaviors in postcoronary patients. *Journal of Psychology, 119*(1), 87–94.

Finney, J., Hook, R., Friman, P., Rapoff, M., & Cage, C. D. (1993). The overestimation of adherence to pediatric medical regimens. *Children's Health Care, 22*(4), 297–304.

Fishbain, D., Goldberg, M., Meagher, B., Steele, R., & Rosomoff, H. (1986). Male and female chronic pain patients categorized by DSM-III psychiatric diagnostic criteria. *Pain, 26*, 181–197.

Fleming, J. E., Offord, D. R., & Boyle, M. H. (1989). Prevalence of childhood and adolescent depression in the community: Ontario child health study. *British Journal of Psychiatry, 155*, 647–654.

Fontaine, R., Ontiveros, A., Elie, R., & V'ezina, M. (1992). Lithium carbonate augmentation of desipramine and fluoxetine in refractory depression. *Biological Psychiatry, 29*(9), 946–948.

Fox, R. E. (1995). The rape of psychotherapy. *Professional Psychology: Research and Practice, 26*(2), 147–155.

Frank, E., & Kupfer, D. (1987). Efficacy of combined imipramine and interpersonal psychotherapy. *Psychopharmacology Bulletin, 23*(1), 4–7.

Frank, E., Kupfer, D., Perel, J., Cornes, C., Jarrett, D., Mallinger, A., Thase, M., & Grochocinski, V. (1990). Three-year outcomes for maintenance therapies in recurrent depression. *Archives of General Psychiatry, 47*, 1093–1099.

Frank, E., Perel, J., Mallinger, A., Thase, M., & Kupfer, D. J. (1992). Relationship of pharmacologic compliance to long-term prophylaxis in recurrent depression. 30th annual meeting of the American College of Neuropsychopharmacology (1991, San Juan, PR). *Psychopharmacology Bulletin, 28*(3), 231–235.

Frank, J. D. (1973). *Persuasion and healing* (2nd ed.). Baltimore: Johns Hopkins University Press.

Frankel, B. L. (1994). Management of the acutely disturbed medical patient in a hospital setting. *Audio-Digest, Psychiatry, 23*(12).

Franks, C. M., & Mays, D. T. (1980). Negative effects revisited: A rejoinder. *Professional Psychology, 11*(1), 101–105.

Freeman, M. A. (1995, March). *A look at the future of managed behavioral healthcare: Trends, implications, and opportunities for CMHCs.* Paper presented at Stragetic Planning Work Days at Spokane Community Health Center, Spokane, WA.

Freeman, T. W., Clothier, J. L., Pazzaglia, P., Lesem, M. D., & Swann, A. L. (1992). A double-blind comparison of valproate and lithium in the treatment of acute mania. *American Journal of Psychiatry, 149*, 108.

Freud, S. (1986). Mourning and melancholia. In J. C. Coyne (Ed.), *Essential papers on depression* (pp. 48–63). New York: New York University Press.

Gallagher, D., & Thompson, L. (1982). Treatment of major depressive disorder in older adult outpatients with brief psychotherapies. *Psychotherapy: Theory, Research, and Practice, 19*(4), 482–490.

Gallagher, D., & Thompson, L. (1983). Effectiveness of psychotherapy for both endogenous and nonendogenous depression in older adult outpatients. *Journal of Gerontology, 38*(6), 707–712.

Gallagher-Thompson, D., Hanley-Peterson, P., & Thompson, L. (1990). Maintenance of gains versus relapse following brief psychotherapy for depression. *Journal of Consulting and Clinical Psychology, 58*(3), 371–374.

Geiselmann, B., & Linden, M. (1991). Prescription and intake patterns in long-term and ultra-long-term benzodiazepine treatment in primary care practice. *Pharmacopsychiatry, 24*(2), 55–61.

Geller, B., Cooper, T. B., McCombs, H. G., Graham, D. L., & Wells, J. (1989). Double-blind placebo-controlled study of nortriptyline in depressed children using a "fixed plasma level" design. *Psychopharmacology Bulletin, 25*, 101–108.

George, M. S. (1993). Brain activation involving mood and mood disorders. *Audio-Digest, Psychiatry, 24*(09).

George, M. S., Ketter, T. A., Parekh, P. I., Aorwitz, B., Herscovitch, P., & Post, R. M. (1995). Brain activity during transient sadness and happiness in healthy women. *American Journal of Psychiatry, 152,* 341.

Georgotas, A., McCue, R. E., & Hapworth, W. (1986). Comparative efficacy and safety of MAOIs vs. TCAs in treating depression in the elderly. *Biological Psychiatry, 21,* 1155–1166.

Gerner, R. H. (1993). The new mood stabilizers. *Audio-Digest, Psychiatry, 22* (13).

Gerner, R. H. (1994). Managing refractory mood disorders. *Audio-Digest, Psychiatry, 23*(07).

Giardina, E. G., Bigger, J. T., Jr., Glassman, A. H., Perel, J. M. & Kantor, S. J. (1979). The electrocardiographic and antiarrhythmic effects of imipramine hydrochloride at therapeutic plasma concentrations. *Circulation, 60,* 1045–1052.

Giblin, P. (1989). Use of reading assignments in clinical practice. *American Journal of Family Therapy, 17*(3), 219–228.

Giles, D., Jarrett, R., Biggs, M., Guzick, D., & Rush A. (1989). Clinical predictors of recurrence in depression. *American Journal of Psychiatry, 146*(6), 764–767.

Glaser, K. (1967). Masked depression in children and adolescents. *American Journal of Psychotherapy, 21,* 565–574.

Glaser, R., Strain, E. C., Tarr, K. L., Holliday, J. E., Donnerberg, R. L., & Kiecolt-Glaser, J. K. (1985). Changes in Epstein-Barr virus antibody titers associated with aging. *Proceedings of the Society for Experimental Biology and Medicine, 179*(3), 352–355.

Glassman, A. H., Bigger, J. T., Jr., Giardina, E. V., & Roose, S. P. (1979). Clinical characteristics of imipramine-induced orthostatic hypotension. *Lancet, 1,* 468–472.

Glassman, A. H., Johnson, L. L., & Giardiana, E. G. V. (1983). The use of imipramine in depressed patients with congestive heart failure. *Journal of the American Medical Association, 250,* 1997–2001.

Gleser, J., & Mendelberg, H. (1990). Exercise and sport in mental health: A review of the literature. *Israel Journal of Psychiatry & Related Sciences, 27*(2), 99–112.

Gold, J. R. (1990). Levels of depression. In B. B. Wolman & G. Stricker (Eds.), *Depressive disorders: Facts, theories, and treatment methods* (pp. 203–228). New York: Wiley.

Goldberg, J. F., Harrow, M., & Grossman, L. S. (1995). Recurrent affective syndromes in bipolar and unipolar mood disorders at follow-up. *British Journal of Psychiatry, 166*(3), 382–385.

Goldberg, R. J. (1995). Diagnostic dilemmas presented by patients with anxiety and depression. *American Journal of Medicine, 98,* 278–284.

Golden, R. N., & Janowsky, D. S. (1990). Biological theories of depression. In B. B. Wolman & G. Stricker (Eds.), *Depressive disorders: Facts, theories, and treatment methods* (pp. 3–21). New York: Wiley.

Goldfried, M. R., & Castonguay, L. G. (1992). The future of psychotherapy integration. *Psychotherapy, 29*(1), 4.

Goodwin, D. W., Schulsinger, F., Hermansen, L., Hermansen, L., Guze, S. B., & Winokur, G. (1973). Alcohol problems in adoptees raised apart from alcoholic biological parents. *Archives of General Psychiatry, 28,* 238–243.

Goodwin, D. W., Schulsinger, F., Knopf, J., Mednick, S., & Guze, S. B. (1977). Psychopathology in adopted and nonadopted daughters of alcoholics. *Archives of General Psychiatry, 34,* 1005–1009.

Goodwin, F. K. (1994). Treatment-resistant bipolar patients. *Audio-Digest, Family Practice, 23*(17).

Goodwin, F. K., & Bunney, W., Jr. (1971). Depressions following reserpine: A reevaluation. *Seminars in Psychiatry, 3*(4), 435–448.

Goodwin, F., & Jamison, K. (1990). Suicide. In A. Roy (Ed.), *Manic Depression* (pp. 227–244). Baltimore, MD: Williams & Wilkins.

Goodwin, F. K., & Moskowitz, J. (1993). *Health care reform for Americans with severe mental illness.* Report of National Advisory Mental Health Council, National Institute of Mental Health, Bethesda, MD.

Gotlib, I. H., & Asarnow, R. F. (1979). Interpersonal and impersonal problem-solving skills in mildly and clinically depressed university students. *Journal of Consulting and Clinical Psychology, 47,* 86–95.

Gotlib, I. H., & Colby, C. A. (1987). *Treatment of depression: An interpersonal systems approach.* New York: Pergamon Press.

Gotlib, I. H., & Hammen, C. L. (1992). *Psychological aspects of depression: Toward a cognitive-interpersonal integration.* New York: Wiley.

Gotlib, I. H., & Lee, C. M. (1989). The social functioning of depressed patients. A longitudinal assessment. *Journal of Social and Clinical Psychology, 8,* 223–237.

Gotlib, I. H., & Robinson, L. A. (1982). Responses to depressed individuals: Discrepancies between self-report and observer-rated behaviour. *Journal of Abnormal Psychology, 91,* 231–240.

Gould, R., & Clum, G. (1993). A meta-analysis of self-help treatment approaches. *Clinical Psychology Review, 13*(2), 169–186.

Gray, J. A. (1987). *The psychology of fear and stress* (2nd ed.). Cambridge, England: Cambridge University Press.

Green, P., Stiglin, L., Finkelstein, S., & Berndt, E. (1993). Depression: A neglected major illness. *Journal of Clinical Psychiatry, 54*(11), 419–424.

Greenbaum, P. E., Prange, M. E., Friedman, R. M., & Silver, S. E. (1991). Substance abuse prevalence and comorbidity with other psychiatric disorders among adolescents with severe emotional disturbances. *Journal of the American Academy of Child Psychiatry, 30,* 575–583.

Greenberg, P., Stiglin, L., Finkelstein, S., & Berndt, E. (1993). The economic burden of depression in 1990. *Journal of Clinical Psychiatry, 54*(11), 405–418.

Grunhaus, L. (1994). Major depressive disorder: The syndrome and its characteristics. In L. Grunhaus & J. F. Greden (Eds.), *Severe depressive disorders* (pp. 159–194). Washington, DC: American Psychiatric Press.

Grunhaus, L., & Greden, J. F. (1994). *Severe depressive disorders.* Washington, DC: American Psychiatric Press.

Grunhaus, L., & Pande, A. C. (1994). Electroconvulsive therapy for severe depressive disorders. In L. Grunhaus & J. F. Greden (Eds.), *Severe depressive disorders* (pp. 297–330). Washington, DC: American Psychiatric Press.

Grunhaus, L., Pande, A. C., & Haskett, R. F. (1990). Full and abbreviated courses of maintenance electrconvulsive therapy. *Convulsive Therapy, 6,* 130–138.

Guilleminault, C. (1993). Amphetamines and narcolepsy: Use of the Stanford database. *Sleep, 16*(3), 199–201.

Gullick E., & King L. (1979). Appropriateness of drugs prescribed by primary care physicians for depressed outpatients. *Journal of Affective Disorders, 1*(1), 55–58.

Guze, G., & Gitlin, M. (1994). New antidepressants and the treatment of depression. *Journal of Family Practice, 38*(1), 49–57.

Hadley, S. W., & Strupp, H. H. (1976). Contemporary views of negative effects in psychotherapy: An integrated account. *Archives of General Psychiatry, 33*(11), 1291–1302.

Hafner, R. (1994). Spouse-aided therapy in psychiatry: An introduction. *Australian/New Zealand Journal of Psychiatry, 15,* 329–337.

Haley, J. (1976). *Problem solving therapy.* San Francisco: Jossey-Bass.

Haley, W., Turner, J., & Romano, J. (1985). Depression in chronic pain patients: Relation to pain, activity, and sex differences. *Pain, 23,* 337–343.

Hall, R., Gardner, E., Stickney, S., LeCann, A., & Popkin, M. (1980). Physical illness manifesting as psychiatric disease: II. Analysis of a state hospital inpatient population. *Archives of General Psychiatry, 37,* 989–995.

Hamilton, M. (1960). A rating scale for depression. *Journal of Neurology, Neurosurgery & Psychiatry, 23,* 56–62.

Hamilton, M. (1968). Development of a rating scale for primary depressive illness. *British Journal of Social and Clinical Psychology, 6,* 278–296.

Hammen, C. L. (1981). Assessment: A clinical and cognitive emphasis. In L. P. Rehm (Ed.), *Behavior therapy for depression: Present status and future directions* (pp. 255–277). New York: Academic Press.

Hammen, C. L., & Peters, S. D. (1978). Interpersonal consequences of depression: Responses to men and women enacting a depressed role. *Journal of Abnormal Psychology, 87,* 322–332.

Hankin, J. R., Kessler, L. G., & Goldberg, I. D. (1983). A longitudinal study of offset in the use of nonpsychiatric services following specialized mental health care. *Medical Care, 21,* 1099–1110.

Harrington, R. (1993). *Depressive disorder in childhood and adolescence.* New York: Wiley.

Harter, S. (1983). Developmental perspectives on the self-system. In P. H. Mussen (Series Ed.) & E. M. Hetherington (Vol. Ed.), *Handbook of child psychology, Vol. 4: Socialization, personality, and social development* (4th ed., pp. 275–385). New York: Wiley.

Hartup, W. (1983). Peer relations. In P. H. Mussen (Series Ed.) & E. M.

Hetherington (Vol. Ed.), *Handbook of child psychology, Vol. 4: Socialization, personality, and social development* (4th ed., pp. 103–196). New York: Wiley.

Hasin, D. S., Endicott, J., & Keller, M. B. (1989). RDC alcoholism in patients with major affective syndromes: Two-year course. Presented at 141st annual meeting of the American Psychiatric Association, Montreal, Canada. *American Journal of Psychiatry, 146*(3), 318–323.

Hasin, D. S., & Grant, B. F. (1987). Diagnosing depressive disorders in patients with alcohol and drug problems: A comparison of the SADS-L and the DIS. *Journal of Psychiatric Research, 21*(3), 301–311.

Hasin, D. S., Grant, B. F., & Endicott, J. (1988). Lifetime psychiatric comorbidity in hospitalized alcoholics: Subject and familiar correlates. *International Journal of Addictions, 23*(8), 827–850.

Hathaway, S. R., & McKinley, J. C. (1942). A multiphasic personality schedule. *Journal of Psychology, 14*, 73–84.

Hawkins, D. R. (1994). Sleep and depression. In V. D. Volkan (Ed.), *Depressive states and their treatment* (pp. 359–379). Northvale, NJ: Jason Aronson.

Hay, D. B. (1993). Electroconvulsive therapy. In J. Sadavoy, L. W. Lazarus, & L. F. Jarvik (Eds.), *Comprehensive review of geriatric psychiatry* (pp. 469–486). Washington, DC: American Psychiatric Press.

Healy, D. (1993). Dysphoria. In C. G. Costello (Ed.), *Symptoms of depression* (pp. 23–42). New York: Wiley.

Hecht, H., von Zerssen, D., & Wittchen, H. (1990). Anxiety and depression in a community sample: The influence of comorbidity on social functioning. *Journal of Affective Disorders, 18*, 137–144.

Hedlund, J., & Vieweg, B. (1979). The Hamilton rating scale for depression: A comprehensive review. *Journal of Operational Psychiatry, 10*, 149–162.

Hellerstein, D. J., Samstag, L. W., Little, S., & Yanowitch, P. (1994, May 21–26). *Dysthymia: Assessing symptoms and treatment response with the Cornell dysthymia rating scale.* Presented at the annual meeting, American Psychiatric Association, Philadelphia, PA. *(New Research Program and Abstracts,* p. 111).

Helzer, J. E., & Pryzbeck, T. R. (1988). The co-occurrence of alcoholism with other psychiatric disorders in the general population and its impact on treatment. *Journal of the Studies of Alcohol, 49*(3), 219–224.

Herskowitz, R. D. (1990). Outward Bound, diabetes and motivation: Experiential education in a wilderness setting. *Diabetic Medicine, 7*(7), 633–638.

Heston, L. L., Garrard, J., Makris, L., Kane, R. L., Cooper, S., Dunham, T., & Zelterman, D. (1992). Inadequate treatment of depressed nursing home elderly. *Journal of the American Geriatrics Society, 40*, 1117–1122.

Hill, E. M., Wilson, A. F., Elston, R. C., & Winokur, G. (1988). Evidence for possible linkage between genetic markers and affective disorders. *Biological Psychiatry, 24*, 903–917.

Hill, M. (1992). Light, circadian rhythms, and mood disorders: A review. *Annals of Clinical Psychiatry, 4*(2), 131–146.

Hinchliffe, M., Hooper, D., & Roberts, F. J. (1978). *The melancholy marriage.* New York: Wiley.

Hinkle, J. S. (1992). Aerobic running behavior and psychotherapeutics: Implications for sports counseling and psychology. *Journal of Sport Behavior, 15*(4), 263–277.

Hodges, K. (1990). Depression and anxiety in children: A comparison of self-report questionnaires to clinical interview. *Psychological Assessment: A Journal of Consulting and Clinical Psychology, 2,* 376–381.

Hodges, K., Kline, J., Stern, L., Cytryn, L., & McKnew, D. (1982). The development of a child assessment interview for research and clinical use. *Journal of Abnormal Child Psychology, 10,* 173–189.

Holister, L. E. (1994). New psychotherapeutic drugs. *Journal of Clinical Psychopharmacology, 14*(1), 50–63.

Holloway, R., Rogers, J., & Gershenhorn, S. (1992). Differences between patient and physician perceptions of predicted compliance. *Family Practice, 9*(3), 318–322.

Holmes, T. H., & Rahe, R. H. (1967). The social readjustment rating scale. *Journal of Psychosomatic Research, 11,* 213–218.

Howard, K. I., Kopta, S. M., Krause, M. J., & Orlinsky, D. E. (1986). The dose-effect relationship in psychotherapy. *American Psychologist, 41,* 159–164.

Hoyt, M. F. (1990). On time in brief therapy. In R. A. Wells & V. J. Giannetti (Eds.), *Handbook of the brief psychotherapies* (pp. 115–144). New York: Plenum Press.

Hudson, J. I., Hudson, M. S., Pliner, L. F., Goldenberg, D. L., & Pope, H. G., Jr. (1985). Fibromyalgia and major affective disorder: A controlled phenomenology and family history study. *American Journal of Psychiatry, 142*(4), 441–446.

Hunt, R. D. (1995). Bupropion. *Audio-Digest, Psychiatry, 24*(07).

Isen, A. M. (1987). Positive affect, cognitive processes and social behavior. In L. Berkowitz (Ed.), *Advances in experimental social psychology* (Vol. 20, pp. 203–253). New York: Academic Press.

Jacobson, S., Fasman, J., & DiMascio, A. (1975). Deprivation in the childhood of depressed women. *The Journal of Nervous and Mental Disease, 160,* 5–14.

Janowsky, D. S., El-Yousef, M. K., Davis, J. M., & Sererke, H. J. (1972). A cholinergic-adrenergic hypothesis of mania and depression. *Lancet, 2,* 6732–6735.

Jansen, M. (1986). Emotional disorders in the labour force: Prevalence, costs, prevention and rehabilitation. *International Labour Review, 125*(5), 605–615.

Jaspers, K. (1968). *General psychopathology* (J. Joenig & M. W. Hamilton, Trans.). Chicago: University of Chicago Press. (Originally published 1913)

Jefferson, J. W. (1995a). Side effects of lithium. *Audio-Digest, Psychiatry, 24*(09).

Jefferson, J. W. (1995b). The new antidepressants. *Audio-Digest, Psychiatry, 24*(13).

Jenkins, J. H., Kleinman, A., & Good, B. J. (1991). Cross-cultural studies of depression. In J. Becker & A. Kleinman (Eds.), *Psychosocial aspects of depression* (pp. 67–99). Hillsdale, NJ: Erlbaum.

Joffe, R. T., Levitt, A. J., Bagby, R. M., MacDonald, C., & Singer, W. (1993). Predictors of response to lithium and triiodothyronine augmentation of antidepressants in tricyclic non-responders. *British Journal of Psychiatry, 163,* 574–578.

Joffe, R. T., & Regan, J. (1988). Personality and depression. *Journal of Psychiatric Research, 22,* 279–286.

Johnson, D. (1974). Study of the use of antidepressant medication in general practice. *British Journal of Psychiatry, 125,* 186–212.

Johnson, J., Weissman, M. M., & Klerman, G. L. (1990). Panic disorder, comorbidity, and suicide attempts. *Archives of General Psychiatry, 47*(9), 805–808.

Kalinowsky, L. B. (1975). Electric and other convulsive treatments. In S. Arieti (Ed.), *American handbook of psychiatry v. treatment* (2nd ed.). New York: Basic Books.

Kamlet, M. S. (1990). *Depression in the workplace: Issues and answers.* Baltimore: NIMH/DART.

Kanfer, F. H. (1977). The many faces of self-control, or behavior modification changes its focus. In R. B. Stuart (Ed.), *Behavioral self-management* (pp. 116–122). New York: Brunner/Mazel.

Karasu, T. B. (1990). *Psychotherapy for depression.* Northvale, NJ: Jason Aronson.

Kashani, J., Holcomb, W. R., & Orvaschel, H. (1986). Depression and depressive symptoms in preschool children from the general population. *American Journal of Psychiatry, 143,* 1138–1143.

Katon, W. J. (1984). Depression: Relationship to somatization and chronic medical illness. *Journal of Clinical Psychiatry, 45*(3, Sec. 2), 4–12.

Katon, W. J. (1985). Somatization in primary care. *Journal of Family Practice, 21*(4), 257–258.

Katon, W. J. (1987). The epidemiology of depression in medical care. *International Journal of Psychiatry Medicine, 17*(1), 93–112.

Katon, W. J. (1988). Depression: Somatization and social factors. *Journal of Family Practice, 27*(6), 579–580.

Katon, W. J. (1993, April 30). Somatization: Its relationship to anxiety, depression and personality disorders. Presented at Mental Health Update, University of Washington, Seattle.

Katon, W. J. (1993, April 30). The development of a randomized trial of consultation-liaison psychiatry trial in distressed high utilizers of primary care. Presented at Mental Health Update, University of Washington, Seattle.

Katon, W. J. (1995, May 5). Roots of somatization 2: Anxiety, depression or personality disorders? Presented at Mental Health Update: *Psyche or soma? Difficult differential diagnoses,* University of Washington, Seattle.

Katon, W. J., Kleinman, A., & Rosen, G. (1982). Depression and somatization: A review. Part I. *American Journal of Medicine, 72*(1), 127–135.

Katon, W. J., Ries, R., & Kleinman, A. (1984). Part III: A prospective DSM-III study of 100 consecutive somatization patients. *Comprehensive Psychiatry, 25,* 305–314.

Katon, W. J., & Russo, J. (1989). Somatic symptoms and depression. *Journal of Family Practice, 29*(1), 65–69.

Katon, W. J., & Sullivan, M. D. (1990). Depression and chronic medical illness. *Journal of Clinical Psychiatry, 51*(6; Suppl.), 3–11.

Katon, W. J., von Korff, M., & Lin, E. (1990). Distressed high utilizers of medical care: DSM-III-R diagnoses and treatment needs. *General Hospital Psychiatry,* *12*(6), 355–362.

Katon, W. J., von Korff, M., Lin, E., Walker, E., Simon, G. E., Bush, T., Robinson, P., & Russo, J. (1995). Collaborative management to achieve treatment guidelines: Impact on depression in primary care. *Journal of the American Medical Association, 273*(13), 1026–1031.

Katona, C. L., Abou-Saleh, M. T., Harrison, D. A., Nairac, B. A., Edwards, D. R., Lock, T., Burns, R. A., & Robertson, M. M. (1995). Placebo-controlled trial of lithium augmentation of fluoxetine and lofepramine [published erratum appears in *Br J Psychiatry* 1995 Apr; *166*(4):544]. *British Journal of Psychiatry, 166*(1), 80–86.

Katona, C. L., et al. (1993). Placebo-controlled trial of lithium augmentation of fluoxetine and lofepramine. *International Clinical Psychopharmacology, 8,* 323.

Katz, G., & Watt, J. (1992). Bibliotherapy: The use of books in psychiatric treatment. *Canadian Journal of Psychiatry, 37*(3), 173–178.

Katzelnick, D. J. (1993). Managing the patient on benzodiazepines. *Audio-Digest, Psychiatry, 22* (18).

Kaufmann, C. (1993). Roles for mental health consumers in self-help group research. Special issue: Advances in understanding with self-help groups. *Journal of Applied Behavioral Science, 29*(2), 257–271.

Kearns, N., Cruickshank, L. A., McGuigan, K. J., Riley, S. A., Shaw, S. P., & Snaith, R. P. (1982). A comparison of depression rating scales. *British Journal of Psychiatry, 141,* 45–49.

Keck, P. (1994). Comorbidity in first-episode mania (FEM) compared with multiple-episode mania (MEM). *Audio-Digest, Psychiatry, 23* (09).

Keitner, G. I., Miller, I. W., & Ryan, C. E. (1994). Family functioning in severe depressive disorders. In L. Grunhaus & J. F. Greden (Eds.), *Severe depressive disorders* (pp. 89–110). Washington, DC: American Psychiatric Press.

Kellner, R. (1991). *Psychosomatic syndromes and somatic symptoms.* Washington, DC: American Psychiatric Press.

Kelly, G. (1955). *The psychology of personal constructs* (Vols. 1 and 2). New York: Norton.

Kendall, P. C., & Clarkin, J. F. (1992). Introduction to special section: Comorbidity and treatment implications. *Journal of Consulting and Clinical Psychology, 60*(6), 833–834.

Kendall, P. C., Stark, K. D., & Adam, T. (1990). Cognitive deficit or cognitive distortion in childhood depression. *Journal of Abnormal Child Psychology, 18,* 255–270.

Kendell, R. E. (1988). What is a case? Food for thought for epidemiologists. *Archives of General Psychiatry, 45,* 374–376.

Kennedy, B. L. (1995). Gender differences and psychopharmacologic agents. *Audio-Digest, Psychiatry, 24* (11).

Kennedy, B. P. (1993). The Beech Hill hospital/Outward Bound adolescent chemical dependency treatment program. *Journal of Substance Abuse Treatment, 10*(4), 395–406.

Kennedy, S., Kiecolt-Glaser, J. K., & Glaser, R. (1988). Immunological consequences of acute and chronic stressors: Mediating role of interpersonal relationships. *British Journal of Medical Psychology, 61*(Pt.1), 77–85.

Kessler, L. G., Cleary, P., & Burke, J. (1985). Psychiatric disorders in primary care. *Archives of General Psychiatry, 42,* 583–587.

Kessler, L. G., Steinwachs, D. M., & Hankin, J. R. (1982). Episodes of psychiatric care and medical utilization. *Medical Care, 20,* 1209–1221.

Kessler, R., (1994). *Prevalence and comorbidity of major psychiatric disorders.* Ann Arbor: University of Michigan Survey Research Center.

Ketter, T. (1995). Anatomy and pharmacology of depression. *Audio-Digest, Psychiatry, 24*(08).

Keys, A. (1950). *The biology of human starvation.* Minneapolis: University of Minnesota Press.

Kiewa, J. (1994). Self-control: The key to adventure? Towards a model of the adventure experience. *Women & Therapy, 15*(3–4), 29–41.

Kirmayer, L. J. (1987). Languages of suffering and healing: Alexithymia as a social and cultural process. *Transcultural Psychiatric Research Review, 24,* 119–136.

Klein, M. (1934). A contribution to the psychogenesis of manic-depressive states. In *Contributions to psycho-analysis, 1921–1945* (pp. 282–310). London: Hogarth Press.

Kleinman, A., & Good, B. (1985). Epilogue. In A. Kleinman & B. Good (Eds.), *Culture and depression: Studies in the anthropology and cross-cultural psychiatry of affect and disorder.* Berkeley: University of California Press.

Klerman, G. L. (1978). Psychopharmacologic treatment of depression. In J. G. Bernstein (Ed.), *Clinical Psychopharmacology* (pp. 63–79). Littleton, MA: PSG Publishing.

Klerman, G. L. (1979). International perspectives of psychopharmacology: The interface of research and treatment. *Psychopharmacology Bulletin, 15*(3), 51–53.

Klerman, G. L., DiMascio, A., Weissman, M., Prusoff, B., & Paykel, E. (1974). Treatment of depression by drugs and psychotherapy. *American Journal of Psychiatry, 131*(2), 186–192.

Klerman, G. L., & Weissman, M. (1987). Interpersonal psychotherapy (IPT) and drugs in the treatment of depression. *Pharmacopsychiatry, 20,* 3–7.

Klerman, G. L., Weissman, M., Rounsaville, B., & Chevron, R. (1984). *Interpersonal psychotherapy of depression.* New York: Basic Books.

Klingle, R. (1993). Bringing time into physician compliance-gaining research: Toward a reinforcement expectancy theory of strategy effectiveness. *Health Communication, 5*(4), 283–308.

Knesper, D. J. (1994). Organic affective syndromes. *Audio-Digest, Psychiatry, 23*(02).

Kogan, L. S. (1957). The short-term case in a family agency: Part III. Further results and conclusion. *Social Casework, 38,* 366–374.

Kornblith, S., Rehm, L., O'Hara, M., & Lamparski, D. (1983). The contribution of self-reinforcement training and behavioral assignments to the efficacy of self-control therapy for depression. *Cognitive Therapy & Research, 7*(6), 499–528.

Kovacs, M. (1981). Rating scales to assess depression in school-aged children. *Acta Paidopsychiatrica, 46*(5–6), 305–315.

Kovacs, M. (1986). A developmental perspective on methods and measures in the assessment of depressive disorders: The clinical interview. In M. Rutter, C. E. Izard, & R. B. Read (Eds.), *Depression in young people: Developmental and clinical perspectives* (pp. 435–465). New York: Guilford Press.

Kovacs, M. (1992). *The children's depression inventory.* New York: Multi-Health Systems.

Kovacs, M., & Beck, A. T. (1986). Maladaptive cognitive structures in depression. In J. C. Coyne (Ed.), *Essential papers on depression* (pp. 240–258). New York: New York University Press.

Kovacs, M., & Paulauskas, S. L. (1984). Developmental state and the expression of depressive disorders in children: An empirical analysis. In D. Cicchetti & K. Schneider-Rosen (Eds.), *New direction for child development: No. 26. Childhood depression* (pp. 59–80). San Francisco: Jossey-Bass.

Kovacs, M., Rush, A., Beck, A., & Hollon, S. (1981). Depressed outpatients treated with cognitive therapy or pharmacotherapy: A one-year follow-up. *Archives of General Psychiatry, 38,* 33–41.

Kramlinger, K., Swanson, D., & Maruta, T. (1983). Are patients with chronic pain depressed? *American Journal of Psychiatry, 140*(6), 747–749.

Kreitman, N. (1977). *Parasuicide.* Chichester, England: Wiley.

Kroll, J., Linde, P., Habenicht, M., Chan, S., Yan, G. M., Van G. T., Souvannasoth, L., Nguyen, J., Ly, T., & Nguyen, H. (1990). Medication compliance, antidepressant blood levels, and side effects in Southeast Asian patients. *Journal of Clinical Psychopharmacology, 10*(4), 279–283.

Kukull, W. A., Koepsell, T. D., Inui, T. S., & Borson, S. (1986). Depression and physical illness among elderly general medical clinic patients. *Journal of Affective Disorders, 10,* 153–162.

Kupfer, D. J., Carpenter, L. L., & Frank, E. (1988). Possible role of antidepressants in precipitating mania and hypomania in recurrent depression. *American Journal of Psychiatry, 145*(7), 804–808.

Kupfer, D. J., Frank, E., & Perel, J. (1989). The advantage of early treatment intervention in recurrent depression. *Archives of General Psychiatry, 46,* 771–775.

Kupfer, D. J., Frank, E., Perel, J., Cornes, C., Mallinger, A., Thase, M., McEachran, A., & Grochocinski, V. (1992). Five-year outcome for maintenance therapies in recurrent depression. *Archives of General Psychiatry, 49,* 769–773.

Lacks, P. (1987). *Behavioral treatment for persistent insomnia.* New York: Pergamon Press.

Large, R. (1986). DSM-III diagnoses in chronic pain. *Journal of Nervous & Mental Disease, 174*(5), 295–303.

Last, C., Thase, M., Hersen, M., Bellack, A., & Himmelhoch, J. (1985). Patterns of attrition for psychosocial and pharmacologic treatments of depression. *Journal of Clinical Psychiatry, 46*(9), 361–366.

Lazarus, A. A. (1968). Learning theory and the treatment of depression. *Behaviour Research and Therapy, 6,* 83–89.

Lechnyr, R. (1992). Cost savings and effectiveness of mental health services. *Journal of the Oregon Psychological Association, 38,* 8–12.

Lecrubier, Y., & Guelfi, J. D. (1990). Efficacy of reversible inhibitors of monoamine oxidase-A in various forms of depression. *Acta Psychiatrica Scandinavica, 360*(Suppl.), 18–23.

Lee, C. (1992). Getting fit: A minimal intervention for aerobic exercise. *Behavior Change, 9*(4), 223–228.

Lee, S. (1993). The prevalence and nature of lithium noncompliance among Chinese psychiatric patients in Hong Kong. *Journal of Nervous & Mental Disease, 181*(10), 618–625.

Lehofer, M., Klebel, H., Gersdorf, C. H., & Zapotoczky, H. G. (1992). Running and motion therapy for depression. 7th Psychiatric Forum: Actual aspect of depression (1991, Salzburg, Austria). *Psychiatria Danubina,* 4(1–2), 149–152.

Lejoyeau, M., Ades, J., & Rouillon, F. (1994). Serotonin syndrome: Incidence, symptoms and treatment. *CNS Drugs, 2*(2), 132–143.

Lenkowsky, R. (1987). Bibliotherapy: A review and analysis of the literature. *Journal of Special Education, 21*(2), 123–132.

Levander, S., & Sachs, C. (1987). Arousal and personality traits: Effects of central stimulants in narcolepsy. *Personality & Individual Differences, 8*(3), 365–370.

Lewinsohn, P. M. (1974). A behavioral approach to depression. In R. J. Friedman & M. M. Katz (Eds.), *The psychology of depression: Contemporary theory and research* (pp. 157–185). New York: Wiley.

Lewinsohn, P. M. (1986). A behavioral approach to depression. In J. C. Coyne (Ed.), *Essential papers on depression* (pp. 150–180). New York: New York University Press.

Lewinsohn, P., Antonuccio, D., Steinmetz, J., & Teri, L. (1984). *The coping with depression course: A psychoeducational intervention for unipolar depression.* Eugene, OR: Castalia Press.

Lewinsohn, P. M., Clarke, G. N., Hops, H., & Andrews, J. (1990). Cognitive-behavioural treatment for depressed adolescents. *Behaviour Therapy, 21,* 385–401.

Lewinsohn, P. M., Hoberman, H. M., & Rosenbaum, M. (1988). A prospective study of risk factors for unipolar depression. *Journal of Abnormal Psychology, 97,* 251–264.

Lewinsohn, P. M., Hoberman, H., Teri, L., & Hautzinger, M. (1985). An integrative theory of depression. In S. Reiss & R. Bootzin (Eds.), *Theoretical issues in behavior therapy* (pp. 331–359). New York: Academic Press.

Lewinsohn, P. M., Hops, H., Roberts, R. E., Seeley, J. R., & Andrews, J. A. (1993). Adolescent psychopathology: I. Prevalence and incidence of depression and other DSM-III-R disorders in high school students [published erratum appears in *J Abnorm Psychol* 1993 Nov; *102*(4):517]. *Journal of Abnormal Psychology, 102*(1), 133–144.

Lewinsohn, P. M., & Libet, J. (1972). Pleasant events, activity schedules and depression. *Journal of Abnormal Psychology, 79,* 291–295.

Lewinsohn, P. M., Muñoz, R. F., Youngren, M. A., & Zeiss, A. M. (1986). *Control your depression.* New York: Fireside.

Lewinsohn, P., & Teri, L. (1982). Selection of depressed and nondepressed subjects on the basis of self-report data. *Journal of Consulting and Clinical Psychology, 50,* 590–591.

Lewis, A. (1967). Melancholia: Historical review. In A. Lewis (Ed.), *The state of psychiatry: Essays and addresses.* New York: Science House.

Lewis, M., & Volkmar, F. R. (1990). *Clinical aspects of child and adolescent development.* Philadelphia: Lea & Febiger.

Lewy, A. J. (1994). Ordering sleep. *Audio-Digest, Family Practice, 23*(14).

Liberman, R. P., DeRisi, W. J., & Mueser, K. T. (1989). *Social skills training for psychiatric patients.* Boston: Allyn & Bacon.

Lieberman, J. A. (1994). Managing side effects and toxicity of antipsychotic drugs. *Audio-Digest, Psychiatry, 23* (18).

Lindsay, P., & Wyckoff, M. (1981). The depression-pain syndrome and its response to antidepressants. *Psychosomatics, 22*(7), 571–577.

Linehan, M. M. (1981). A social–behavioral analysis of suicide and parasuicide: Implications for clinical assessment and treatment. In H. Glaezer & J. F. Clarkin (Eds.), *Depression: Behavioral and directive intervention strategies* (pp. 279–294). New York: Garland.

Linehan, M. M. (1993). *Cognitive-behavioral treatment of borderline personality disorder.* New York: Guilford Press.

Linnoila, M., Virkkunen, M., Scheinin, M., Nuutila, A., Rimon, R., & Goodwin, F. K. (1983). Low cerebrospinal fluid 5-hydroxyindoleacetic acid concentration differentiates impulsive from nonimpulsive violent behavior. *Life Sciences, 33*, 2609–2614.

Littlepage, G. E., Kosloski, K. D., Schnelle, J. F., McNees, M. P., & Gendrich, J. C. (1976). The problem of early outpatient terminations from community mental health centers: A problem for whom? *Journal of Community Psychology, 4*, 164–167.

Locke, S. E., Kraus, L., Leserman, J., Hurst, M. W., Heisel, J. S., & Williams, R. M. (1984). Life change stress, psychiatric symptoms, and natural killer cell activity. *Psychosomatic Medicine, 46*(5), 441–453.

Lombardi, K. L. (1990). Depressive states and somatic symptoms. In B. B. Wolman & G. Stricker (Eds.), *Depressive disorders: Facts, theories, and treatment methods* (pp. 149–161). New York: Wiley.

Loosen, P. T., Dew, B. W., & Prange, A. J. (1990). Long-term predictors of outcome in abstinent alcoholic men. *American Journal of Psychiatry, 147*, 162–166.

Lowman, R. L., & Resnick, R. J. (1994). *The mental health professional's guide to managed care.* Washington, DC: American Psychological Association.

Luborsky, L., Crits-Christoph, P., Alexander, L., Margolis, M., & Cohen, M. (1983). Two helping alliance methods for predicting outcomes of psychotherapy. *The Journal of Nervous and Mental Disease, 171*, 480–491.

Luborsky, L., Singer, B., & Luborsky, L. (1975). Comparative studies of psychotherapies: Is it true that "everyone has won and all must have prizes"? *Archives of General Psychiatry, 32*, 995–1008.

Ludwigsen, K., & Enright, M. (1988). The health care revolution: Implications for psychology and hospital practice. *Psychotherapy, 25*, 424–428.

Luke, D., Roberts, L., & Rappaport, J. (1993). Individual–group context, and individual–group fit predictors of self-help group attendance. *Journal of Applied Behavioral Science, 29*(2), 216–238.

Lydiard, R. B. (1993). Drugs for depression: The battle of the selective serotonin reuptake inhibitors (SSRIs). *Audio-Digest, Psychiatry, 22*(19).

Lydiard, R. B. (1995a). Some new anxiolytics. *Audio-Digest, Psychiatry, 24*(14).

Lydiard, R. B. (1995b). The new anxiolytics. *Audio-Digest, Psychiatry, 24*(13).

Lynch, D., Birk, T., Weaver, M., Gohara, A., Leighton, R. F., Repka, F. J. & Walsh, M. E. (1992). Adherence to exercise interventions in the treatment of hypercholesterolemia. *Journal of Behavorial Medicine, 15*(40), 365–377.

MacMahon, J. R. (1990). The psychological benefits of exercise and the treatment of delinquent adolescents. *Sports Medicine, 9*(6), 334–351.

Magni, G. (1991). The use of antidepressants in the treatment of chronic pain. A review of the current evidence. *Drugs, 42*(5), 730–748.

Magni, G., Schifano, F., & de Leo, D. (1985). Pain as a symptom in elderly depressed patients: Relationship to diagnostic subgroups. *Archives of Psychiatry and Neurological Science, 235*(3), 143–145.

Magruder-Habib, K., Zung, W., Feussner, J., Alling, W., Saunders, W., & Stevens, H. (1989). Management of general medical patients with symptoms of depression. *General Hospital Psychiatry, 11*, 201–206.

Mahalik, J., & Kivlighan, D. (1988). Self-help treatment for depression: Who succeeds? *Journal of Counseling Psychology, 35*(3), 237–242.

Malan, D. H. (1963). *A study of brief psychotherapy*. New York: Plenum Press.

Malan, D. H (1976). *The frontier of brief psychotherapy*. New York: Plenum Press.

Manaster, G. J., & Corsini, R. J. (1982). *Individual psychology: Theory and practice*. Itasca, IL: Peacock.

Mann, J. (1973). *Time-limited psychotherapy*. Cambridge, MA: Harvard University Press.

Mann, J. (1981). The core of time-limited psychotherapy: Time and the central issue. In S. H. Budman (Ed.), *Forms of brief therapy* (pp. 25–44). New York: Guilford Press.

Margo, G., Dewan, M., Fisher, S., & Greenberg, R. (1992). Comparison of three depression rating scales. *Perceptual & Motor Skills, 75*(1), 144–146.

Markowitz, J. C., & Kocsis, J. H. Dysthymia. (1994). In L. Grunhaus & J. F. Greden (Eds.), *Severe depressive disorders* (pp. 209–222). Washington, DC: American Psychiatric Press.

Markowitz, J. S., Weissman, M. M., Oullette, R., Lish, J. D., & Klerman, G. L. (1989). Quality of life in panic disorder. *Archives of General Psychiatry, 46*, 984–992.

Marks, T., & Hammen, C. L. (1982). Interpersonal mood induction: Situational and individual determinants. *Motivation and Emotion, 6*, 387–399.

Marsella, J., Hirschfeld, R., & Katz, M. (1987). *The measurement of depression*. New York: Guilford Press.

Marsh, H. W., & Richards, G. E. (1986). The Rotter locus of control scale: The comparison of alternative response formats and implications for reliability, validity, and dimensionality. *Journal of Research in Personality, 20*(4), 509–528.

Marsh, H. W., & Richards, G. E. (1988). The Outward Bound bridging course for low-achieving high school males: Effect on academic achievement and multidimensional self-concepts. *Australian Journal of Psychology, 40*(3), 281–298.

Martin, J. E., & Dubbert, P. M. (1982). Exercise and health: The adherence problem. *Behavioral Medicine Update, 4*(1), 16–24.

Maruta, T., Vatterott, M., & McHardy, M. (1989). Pain management as an anti-depressant: Long-term resolution of pain-associated depression. *Pain, 36,* 335–337.

Marx, J., Gyorky, Z., Royalty, G., & Stern. T. (1992). Use of self-help books in psychotherapy. *Professional Psychology: Research and Practice, 23*(4), 300–305.

Matinsen, E. W., & Medhus, A. (1989). Adherence to exercise and patients' evaluation of physical exercise in a comprehensive treatment programme for depression. *Nordisk Psykiatrisk Tidsskrift, 43*(5), 411–415.

Matson, J. L. (1989). *Treating depression in children and adolescents.* New York: Pergamon.

Maultsby, M. (1974). Dream changes following successful rational behavior therapy. *Rational Living, 9*(2), 30–33.

Max, M. B., Lynch, S. A., Muir, J., Shoaf, S. E., Smoller, B., & Dubner, R. (1992). Effects of desipramine, amitriptyline, and fluoxetine on pain in diabetic neuropathy. *New England Journal of Medicine, 326*(19), 1250–1256.

Mays, M. (1979, October). *Cooperative health plan, mental health system design.* Audio cassette recording presented at Mental Health Services in Health Maintenance Organizations, a conference of the Group Health Association of America, Dallas, TX.

Mays, M. (1979). *Developing mental health service.* Proceedings of the Medical Directors Conference, Group Health Association of America, *4*(2), 56–76.

McCauley, E., & Myers, K. (1992). The longitudinal clinical course of depression in children and adolescents. *Mood Disorders, 1*(1), 183–196.

McClelland, D. C. (1961). *The achieving society.* Princeton, NJ: Van Nostrand.

McGee, R., Williams, S., Kashani, J. H., & Silva, P. A. (1983). Prevalence of self-reported depressive symptoms and associated social factors in mothers in Dunedin. *British Journal of Psychiatry, 143,* 473–479.

McLean, P. D., & Hakstian, A. R. (1979). Clinical depression: Comparative efficacy of outpatient treatments. *Journal of Consulting and Clinical Psychology, 47,* 818–836.

McLean, P., Ogston, K., & Grauer, L. (1973). A behavioral approach to the treatment of depression. *Journal of Behavior Therapy and Experimental Psychiatry, 4,* 323–330.

Mc Mullin, R. E. (1986). *Handbook of cognitive therapy techinques.* New York: Norton.

Meats, P., Hellewell, J., & Jolley, D. (1992). Interaction between narcolepsy-cataplexy and bipolar mood disorder in an elderly woman. *International Journal of Geriatric Psychiatry, 7*(2), 135–137.

Meichenbaum, D. (1977). *Cognitive-behavior modification: An integrative approach.* New York: Plenum.

Meichenbaum, D. (1985). *Stress inoculation training.* New York: Pergamon Press.

Merritt, S. L., Cohen, F. L., & Smith, K. M. (1992). Depressive symptomatology in narcolepsy. *Loss, Grief & Care, 5*(3–4), 53–59.

Messiha, F. S. (1993). Fluoxetine: A spectrum of clinical applications and postulates of underlying mechanisms. *Neuroscience and Biobehavioral Reviews, 17*(4), 385–396.

Miklowitz, D. (1992). Longitudinal outcome and medication noncompliance among manic patients with and without mood-incongruent psychotic features. *Journal of Nervous & Mental Disease, 180*(11), 703–711.

Milin, R., Halikas, J. A., Meller, J. E., & Morse, C. (1991). Psychopathology among substance abusing juvenile offenders. *Journal of the American Academy of Child Psychiatry, 30,* 569–574.

Miller, W. R., Rosellini, R. A., & Seligman, E. P. (1986). Learned helplessness and depression. In J. C. Coyne (Ed.), *Essential papers on depression* (pp. 181–219). New York: New York University Press.

Millon, T. (1983). *Millon Clinical Multiaxial Inventory Manual* (3rd ed.). Minneapolis, MN: Interpretive Scoring Systems.

Mintz, J., Mintz, L., Arruda, M., & Hwant, S. (1992). Treatments of depression and the functional capacity to work. *Archives of General Psychiatry, 49*(10), 761–768.

Mitchell, J., McCauley, E., Burke, P., & Moss, S. J. (1988). Phenomenology of depression in children and adolescents. *Journal of the American Academy of Child Psychiatry, 27,* 12–20.

Mitler, M. M., Hajdukovic, R., & Erman, M. K. (1993). Treatment of narcolepsy with methamphetamine. *Sleep, 16*(4), 306–317.

Mitler, M. M., Nelson, S., & Hajdukovic, R. (1987). Narcolepsy: Diagnosis, treatment, and management. *Psychiatric Clinics of North America, 10*(4), 593–606.

Monahan, J., & Steadman, H. J. (1994). *Violence and mental disorder: Developments in risk assessment.* Chicago: University of Chicago Press.

Monroe, S. M., & Depue, R. A. (1991). Life stress and depression. In J. Becker & A. Kleinman (Eds.), *Psychosocial aspects of depression* (pp. 101–130). Hillsdale, NJ: Erlbaum.

Monroe, S. M., Imhoff, D. F., Wise, B. D., & Harris, J. E. (1983). Prediction of psychological symptoms under high risk psychosocial circumstances: Life events, social support and symptom specificity. *Journal of Abnormal Psychology, 92,* 338–350.

Montgomery, S. A., & Asberg, M. C. (1979). A new depression scale designed to be sensitive to change. *British Journal of Psychiatry, 134,* 382–389.

Moos, R. H. (1991). Life stressors, social resources, and the treatment of depression. In J. Becker & A. Kleinman (Eds.), *Psychosocial aspects of depression* (pp. 187–214). Hillsdale, NJ: Erlbaum.

Moreau, D., Mufson, L., Weissman, M. M., & Klerman, G. L. (1991). Interpersonal psychotherapy for adolescent depression: Description of modification and preliminary application. *Journal of the American Academy of Child Psychiatry, 30,* 642–651.

Moretti, M. M., Fine, S., Haley, G., & Marriage, K. (1985). Childhood and adolescent depression: Child-report versus parent-report information. *Journal of the American Academy of Child Psychiatry, 24,* 298–302.

Morton, N. E. (1955). Sequential tests for the detection of linkage. *American Journal of Human Genetics, 7,* 277–318.

Mosak, H. H. (1971). Lifestyle. In A. Nikelly (Ed.), *Techniques for behavior change* (pp. 77–81). Springfield, IL: Charles C. Thomas.

Munjack, D. J., & Moss, H. B. (1981). Affective disorder and alcoholism. *Archives of General Psychiatry, 38,* 869–871.

Murphy, G., Simmons, A., Wetzel, R., & Lustman, P. (1984). Cognitive therapy and notriptyline, singly and together, in the treatment of depression. *Archives of General Psychiatry, 41,* 33–41.

Murphy, P. M., & Kupshik, G. A. (1992). *Loneliness, stress and well-being: A helper's guide.* New York: Routledge.

Myers, E., & Branthwaite, A. (1992). Out-patient compliance with antidepressant medication. *British Journal of Psychiatry, 160,* 83–86.

Myers, E., & Calvert, E. (1984). Information, compliance and side-effects: A study of patients on antidepressant medication. *British Journal of Clinical Pharmacology, 17,* 21–25.

Myers, K. M., & Croake, J. W. (1993). Major depressive disorder during childhood. In L. Sperry & J. Carlson (Eds.), *Psychopathology and psychotherapy: From diagnosis to treatment* (pp. 457–508). Muncie, IN: Accelerated Development.

Narrow, W. E., Regier, D. A., & Rae, D. S. (1993). Use of services by persons with mental and addictive disorders: Findings from the National Institute of Mental Health. *Archives of General Psychiatry, 50*(2), 95–107.

Neimeyer, R., & Feixas, G. (1990). The role of homework and skill acquisition in the outcome of group cognitive therapy for depression. *Behavior Therapy, 21,* 281–292.

Nezu, A. M. (1986). Efficacy of a social problem-solving therapy for unipolar depression. *Journal of Consulting and Clinical Psychology, 54,* 196–202.

Nezu, A. M. (1987). A problem-solving formulation of depression: A literature review and proposal of a pluralistic model. *Clinical Psychology Review, 7,* 121–144.

Nezu, A.M., & Perri, M. (1989). Social problem-solving therapy for unipolar depression: An initial dismantling investigation. *Journal of Consulting and Clinical Psychology, 57*(3), 408–413.

Nierenberg, A. A. (1995). Overcoming treatment-resistant depression. *Audio-Digest, Psychiatry, 24* (14).

NIMH Consensus Development Conference Statement. (1985). Mood disorders: Pharmacologic prevention of recurrences. *American Journal of Psychiatry, 142,* 469–476.

Nofzinger, E. A., Thase, M. E., Reynolds, C. F., Himmelhoch, J. M., Mallinger, A., Houck, P., & Kupfer, D. J. (1991). Hypersomnia in bipolar depression: A comparison with narcolepsy using the multiple sleep latency test. *American Journal of Psychiatry, 148*(9), 1177–1181.

Norcross, J., Alford, B., & DeMichele, J. (1992). The future of psychotherapy: Delphi data and concluding observations. *Psychotherapy, 29*(1), 150–158.

Novak, B. J., Zall, H., & Zavodnick, S. (1994). Somatic treatment of depression. In V. D. Volkan (Ed.), *Depressive states and their treatment* (pp. 401–444). Northvale, NJ: Jason Aronson.

O'Boyle, M., & Hirschfeld, R. M. A. (1994). Recurrent depression: Comorbidity with personality disorder or alcoholism, and impact on quality of life. In L.

Grunhaus & J. F. Greden (Eds.), *Severe depressive disorders* (pp. 141–158). Washington, DC: American Psychiatric Press.

O'Brien, M., Petrie, K., & Raeburn, J. (1992). Adherence to medication regimens: Updating a complex medical issue. *Medical Care Review, 49*(4), 435–454.

O'Hara, M., & Rehm, L. (1983). Hamilton rating scale for depression: Reliability and validity of judgments of novice rates. *Journal of Consulting & Clinical Psychology, 51*, 318.

Oldham, J. M., Skodol, A. E., Kellman, H. D., Hyler, S. E., Rosnick, L., & Davies, M. (1992). Diagnosis of DSM-III-R personality disorders by two structured interviews: Patterns of comorbidity. *American Journal of Psychiatry, 149*(2), 213–220.

Onghena, P., DeCuyper, H., VanHoudenhove, B., & Verstraeten, D. (1993). Mianserin and chronic pain: A double-blind placebo-controlled process and outcome study. *Acta Psychiatrica Scandinavica, 88*(3), 198–204.

Onofrj, M., Curatola, L., Ferracci, F., & Fulgente, T. (1992). Narcolepsy associated with primary temporal lobe B-cells lymphoma in a HLA DR2 negative subject. *Journal of Neurology, Neurosurgery & Psychiatry, 55*(9), 852–853.

Ontiveros, A., Fontaine, R., & Elie, R. (1991). Refractory depression: The addition of lithium to fluoxetine or desipramine. *Acta Psychiatrica Scandinavica, 83*(3), 188–192.

Oren, D., & Rosenthal, N. (1992). Seasonal affective disorders. In E. Paykel (Ed.), *Handbook of affective disorders.* (2nd ed., pp. 551–567). London: Churchill Livingstone.

Orrel, M., & Bebbington, P. (1995). Life events and senile dementia: Affective symptoms. *British Journal of Psychiatry, 166*, 613–620.

Osser, D. N. (1993). A systematic approach to the classification and pharmacotherapy of nonpyschotic major depression and dysthymia. *Journal of Clinical Psychopharmacology, 13*(2), 133–144.

O'Sullivan, K., Rynne, C., Miller, J., O'Sullivan, S., Fitzpatrick, V., Hux, M., Cooney, J., & Clare, A. (1988). A follow-up study of alcoholics with and without coexisting affective disorder. *British Journal of Psychiatry, 152*, 813–819.

Page, C., Benaim, S., & Lappin, F. (1987). A long-term retrospective follow-up study of patients treated with prophylactic lithium carbonate. *British Journal of Psychiatry, 150*, 175–179.

Palmore, E., & Kivett, V. (1977). Changes in life satisfaction: A longitudinal study of persons aged 46–70. *Journal of Gerontology, 32*, 311–316.

Pande, A. C. (1994). Pharmacotherapy of depressive disorders. In L. Grunhaus & J. F. Greden (Eds.), *Severe depressive disorders* (pp. 243–267). Washington, DC: American Psychiatric Press.

Pardeck, J. (1991). Using books in clinical practice. *Psychotherapy in Private Practice, 9*(3), 105–119.

Partonen, T., & Lonnqvist, J. (1993). Effects of light on mood. *Annals of Medicine, 25*(4), 301–302.

Partonen, T., Partonen, M., & Lonnqvist, J. (1993). Frequencies of seasonal major depressive symptoms at high latitudes. *European Archives of Psychiatry & Clinical Neuroscience, 243*(3–4), 189–192.

Pate, R. R., Pratt, M., Blair, S. N., Haskell, W. L., Macera C. A., Bouchard, L., Buchner, D., Ettinger, W., Heath, G. W., & King, A. L. (1995). Physical activity and public health: A recommendation from the Centers of Disease Control and Prevention and the American College of Sports Medicine. *Journal of the American Medical Association, 273*, 402–407.

Pattison, E. M., de Francisco, D., Wood, P., Frazier, H., & Crowder, J. (1975). A psychosocial kinship model for family therapy. *American Journal of Psychiatry, 132*, 1246–1251.

Patton, G. C. (1993). Eating problems. In C. G. Costello (Ed.), *Symptoms of depression* (pp. 227–242). New York: Wiley.

Paykel, E. S., Myers, J. K., Dinelt, M. N., Klerman, G. L., Lindenthal, J. J., & Pepper, M. P. (1969). Life events and depression: A controlled study. *Archives of General Psychiatry, 21*, 753–760.

Peet, M., & Harvey, N. S. (1991). Lithium maintenance: 1. A standard education programme for patients. *British Journal of Psychiatry, 158*, 197–200.

Pennebaker, J. W. (1985). Traumatic experience and psychosomatic disease: Exploring the roles of behavioural inhibition, obsession, and confiding. *Canadian Journal of Psychology, 26*, 82–95.

Pennebaker, J. W., & O'Heeron, R. C. (1984). Confiding in others and illness rate among spouses of suicide and accidental-death victims. *Journal of Abnormal Psychology, 93*, 473–476.

Perri, M., McAdoo, W., Spevak, P., & Newlin, D. (1984). Effect of a multicomponent maintenance program on long-term weight loss. *Journal of Consulting and Clinical Psychology, 52*(3), 480–481.

Petty, F. (1992). The depressed alcoholic: Clinical features and medical management. *General Hospital Psychiatry, 14*, 458–464.

Philipp, M., & Fickinger, M. (1993). Psychotropic drugs in the management of chronic pain syndromes. *Pharmacopsychiatry, 26*(6), 221–234.

Pope, H. G., Jr., Hudson, J. I., Jonas, J. M., & Yurgelun-Todd, D. (1983). Bulimia treated with imipramine: A placebo-controlled, double-blind study. *American Journal of Psychiatry, 140*, 554–558.

Poppen, R. (1988). *Behavioral relaxation training and assessment.* New York: Pergamon Press.

Post, R. M. (1994). Mechanisms underlying the evolution of affective disorders: Implications for long-term treatment. In L. Grunhaus & J. F. Greden (Eds.), *Severe depressive disorders* (pp. 23–65). Washington, DC: American Psychiatric Press.

Post, R. M. (1995). Impact of illness variables on gene expression. *Audio-Digest, Psychiatry, 24*(08).

Powell, T. (1993). Self-help research and policy issues. *Journal of Applied Behavioral Science, 29*(2), 151–165.

Powell, T., & Cameron, M. (1991). Self-help research and the public mental health system. *American Journal of Community Psychology, 19*(5), 797–805.

Poynter, W. L. (1994). *The preferred provider's handbook: Building a successful private therapy practice in the managed care marketplace.* New York: Brunner/Mazel.

Prien, R., & Kupfer, D. (1986). Continuation drug therapy for major depressive episodes: How long should it be maintained? *American Journal of Psychiatry, 143,* 18–23.

Puig-Antich, J., Blau, S., Marx, N., Greenhill, L. L., & Chambers, W. (1978). Prepubertal major depressive disorder: A pilot study. *Journal of the American Academy of Child Psychiatry, 17,* 695–707.

Puig-Antich, J., & Gittelman, R. (1982). Depression in childhood and adolescence. In E. S. Paykel (Ed.), *Handbook of affective disorders* (pp. 379–392). Edinburgh: Churchill Livingstone.

Puig-Antich, J., Perel, J. J., Lupatkin, W., Chambers, W. J., Tabrizi, M. A., King, J., Goetz, R., Davies, M., & Stiller, R. L. (1987). Imipramine in prepubertal major depressive disorders. *Archives of General Psychiatry, 44,* 81–89.

Putnam, D., Finney, J., Barkley, P., & Bonner, M. (1994). Enhancing commitment improves adherence to a medical regimen. *Journal of Consulting and Clinical Psychology 62*(1), 191–194.

Quackenbush, R. (1991). The prescription of self-help books by psychologists: A bibliography of selected bibliotherapy resources. *Psychotherapy, 28*(4), 671–677.

Quinnett, P. G. (1987). *Suicide: The forever decision.* New York: Crossroad Publishing.

Quinnett, P. G. (1992). *Suicide: Intervention and therapy.* Spokane, WA: Classic Publishing.

Radloff, L. (1975). Sex differences in depression: The effects of occupation and marital status. *Sex Roles, 1,* 249–265.

Radloff, L. (1977). The CED-D scale: A self-report depression scale for research in the general population. *Applied Psychological Measurement, 1,* 358–401.

Rado, S. (1928). The problem of melancholia. *International Journal of Psychoanalysis, 9,* 420–438.

Rank, O. (1947). *Will therapy: An analysis of the therapeutic process in terms of relationship.* New York: Knopf.

Rappeport, J. R. (1994). Testifying at deposition and trial. *Audio-Digest, Psychiatry, 23*(12).

Rapport, D. J., & Calabrese, J. R. (1993). Tolerance to fluoxetine. *Journal of Clinical Psychopharmacology, 13*(5), 361.

Raps, C. S., Peterson, C., Reinhard, K. E., Abramson, L. Y., & Seligman, M. E. P. (1982). Attributional style among depressed patients. *Journal of Abnormal Psychology, 91,* 102–108.

Raschka, L. B. (1984). Sleep and violence. *Canadian Journal of Psychiatry, 29*(2), 132–134.

Raskin, A., Boothe, H. H., Reatig, N. A., Schulterbrandt, J. G., & Odle, D. (1971). Factor analyses of normal and depressed patients' memories of parental behavior. *Psychological Reports, 29,* 871–879.

Raskind, M. A. (1993, April 30). *Advances in geriatric psychiatry.* Presented at Mental Health Update, University of Washington, Seattle.

Rehm, L. P. (1977). A self-control model of depression. *Behavior Therapy, 8,* 787–804.

Rehm, L. P. (1979). *Behavior therapy for depression.* New York: Academic Press.

Rehm, L. P. (1986). A self-control model of depression. In J. C. Coyne (Ed.), *Essential papers on depression* (pp. 220–239). New York: New York University Press.

Rehm, L. P., Kaslow, N., & Rabin, A. (1987). Cognitive and behavioral targets in a self-control therapy program for depression. *Journal of Consulting and Clinical Psychology, 55*(1), 60–67.

Rehm, L. P., Kornblith, S., O'Hara, M., Lamparsky, D., Romano, J., & Volkin, J. (1981). An evaluation of major components in a self-control behavior therapy program for depression. *Behavior Modification, 5,* 459–489.

Reynolds, C. F., Frank, E., Perel, J. M., Imber, S. D., Cornes, C., Morycz, R. K., Mazumdar, S., Miller, M. D., Pollock, B. G., Rifai, A. H., & Raskin, M. A. (1992). Combined pharmacotherapy and psychotherapy in the acute and continuation treatment of elderly patients with recurrent major depression: A preliminary report. *American Journal of Psychiatry, 149*(12), 1687–1692.

Reynolds, R. D. (1994). Limbic system dysfunction. *Audio-Digest, Family Practice, 42*(04).

Reynolds, W. M., & Coats, K. I. (1986). A comparison of cognitive-behavioral therapy and relaxation training for the treatment of depression in adolescents. *Journal of Consulting and Clinical Psychology, 54,* 653–660.

Reynolds, W. M., & Stark, K. D. (1987). School-based intervention strategies for the treatment of depression in children and adolescents. In S. G. Forman (Ed.), *School-based affective and social interventions* (pp. 69–88). New York: Haworth Press.

Rice, D. R., Kelman, S., Miller, L. S., & Dunmeyer, S. (1990). *The economic costs of alcohol and drug abuse and mental illness: 1985.* Report submitted to the Office of Financing and Coverage Policy of the Alcohol, Drug Abuse, and Mental Health Administration, U.S. Department of Health and Human Services. San Francisco: Institute for Health and Aging, University of California.

Rich, C., Young, D., & Fowler, R. (1986). San Diego suicide study, I: Young vs. old subjects. *Archives of General Psychiatry, 43,* 577–582.

Rich, C. L., Young, J. G., Fowler, R. C., Wagner, J., & Black, N. A. (1990). Guns and suicide: Possible effects of some specific legislation. *American Journal of Psychiatry, 147*(3), 342–346.

Richelson, E. (1994). Pharmacology of antidepressants—characteristics of the ideal drug. *Mayo Clinic Proceedings, 69,* 1069–1081.

Rie, H. E. (1966). Depression in childhood: A survey of some pertinent contributions. *Journal of the American Academy of Child Psychiatry, 5,* 653–685.

Riordan, R., & Wilson, L. Bibliotherapy: Does it work? *Journal of Counseling & Development, 67*(9), 506–508.

Robins, L. N., Helzer, J. E., Weissman, M. M., Orvaschel, H., Gruenberg, E., Burke, J. D., & Regier, D. A. (1984). Lifetime prevalence of specific psychiatric disorders in three sites. *Archives of General Psychiatry, 41,* 949–958.

Rochlin, G. (1959). The loss complex. *Journal of the American Psychoanalytic Association, 7,* 299–316.

Rohde, P., Lewinsohn, P. M., & Seeley, J. R. (1991). Comorbidity of unipolar depression. II: Comorbidity with other mental disorders in adolescents and adults. *Journal of Abnormal Psychology, 100,* 214–222.

Roose, S. P., Glassman, A. H., & Giardina, E. G. V. (1987). Cardiovascular effects of imipramine and bupropion in depressed patients with congestive heart failure. *Journal of Clinical Psychopharmacology, 7,* 247–251.

Rosen, G. M. (1993). Self-help or hype? Comments on psychology's failure to advance self-care. *Professional Psychology: Research and Practice, 24*(3), 340–345.

Rosen, L., Targum, S., Teman, M., Bryant, M., Hoffman, H., Kasper, S., Hamovit, J., Docherty, J., Welch, B., & Rosenthal, N. (1990). Prevalence of seasonal affective disorder at four latitudes. *Psychiatry Research, 31,* 131–144.

Rosenthal, N., Levendosky, A., Skwerer, R., Joseph-Vanderpool, J., Kelly, K., Hardin, T., Kasper, S., DePlabela, P., & Wehr, T. (1990). Effects of light treatment on core body temperature in seasonal affective disorder. *Biological Psychiatry, 27,* 39–50.

Ross, C. A., & Pam, A. (1995). *Pseudoscience in biological psychiatry: Blaming the body.* New York: Wiley.

Roth, B., Faber, J., Nevsimalova, S., & Tosovsky, J. (1971). The influence of imipramine, dexphenmetrazine and amphetamine sulphate upon the clinical and polygraphic picture of narcolepsy-cataplexy. *Schweizer Archiv für Neurologie, Neurochirurgie und Psychiatrie, 108*(2), 251–260.

Roth, B., & Nevsimalova, S. (1975). Depression in narcolepsy and hypersomnia. *Schweizer Archiv für Neurologie, Neurochirurgie und Psychiatrie, 116*(2), 291–300.

Rothner, A. D. (1995). Teenage headaches. *Audio-Digest, Psychiatry, 24*(12).

Rothschild, A. J., & Schatzberg, A. F. (1994). Diagnosis and treatment of psychotic (delusional) depression. In L. Grunhaus & J. F. Greden (Eds.), *Severe depressive disorders* (pp. 195–207). Washington, DC: American Psychiatric Press.

Rovner, B. W., German, P. S., Brant, L. J., Clark, R., Burton, L., & Folstein, M. F. (1991). Depression and mortality in nursing homes. *Journal of the American Medical Association, 265*(8), 993–996.

Roy, A. (1994). Suicide. In L. Grunhaus & J. F. Greden (Eds.), *Severe depressive disorders* (pp. 223–241). Washington, DC: American Psychiatric Press.

Rubin, R. T. (1990) Mood changes during adolescence. In J. Bancroft & J. Reinisch (Eds.), *Adolescence and puberty.* Oxford: Oxford University Press.

Rude, S. (1986). Relative benefits of assertion or cognitive self-control treatment for depression as a function of proficiency in each domain. *Journal of Consulting and Clinical Psychology, 54*(3), 390–394.

Rudolph, B. A. (1993). The importance of the midpoint review in time-limited therapies. *Professional Psychology: Research and Practice, 24*(3), 346–352.

Rush, A. (1986). Pharmacotherapy and psychotherapy. In L. Derogatis (Ed.), *Clinical psychopharmacology* (pp. 46–67). Menlo Park, CA: Addison-Wesley.

Rush, A. (1988). Cognitive approaches to adherence. In A. Frances & R. Hales

(Eds.), *Annual review of psychiatry* (Vol. 7, pp. 625–640). Washington, DC: American Psychiatric Press.

Rush, A., Beck, A., Kovacs, M., & Hollon, S. (1977). Comparative efficacy of cognitive therapy and pharmacotherapy in the treatment of depressed out-patients. *Cognitive Therapy & Research, 1*, 17–37.

Rush, A. J., Giles, D. E., Schlesser, M. A., Fulton, C. L., Weissenburger, J., & Burns, C. (1986). The inventory for depressive symptomatology (IDS): Preliminary findings. *Psychiatry Research, 18*, 65–87.

Rush, A. J., Shaw, B. F., & Khatami, M. (1980). Cognitive therapy for depression: Utilizing the couples system. *Cognitive Therapy and Research, 4*, 103–113.

Rutter, M. (1986). The developmental psychopathology of depression: Issues and perspectives. In M. Rutter, C. E. Izard, & P. B. Read (Eds.), *Depression in young people: Developmental and clinical perspectives* (pp. 3–30). New York: Guilford Press.

Rutter, M., Tizard, J., & Whitmore, K. (1970). *Education, health and behaviour.* London: Longman.

Ryan, N. D., Puig-Antich, J., Ambrosini, P., Rabinovich, H., Robinson, D., Nelson, B., Iyengar, S., & Twomey, J. (1987). The clinical picture of major depression in children and adolescents. *Archives of General Psychiatry, 44*, 854–861.

Sachs, G. (1995). Overcoming treatment-resistant bipolar disorder. *Audio-Digest, Psychiatry, 24* (11).

Salzman, C. (1976). Interpersonal problems in narcolepsy. *Psychosomatics, 17*(1), 49–51.

Salzman, C. (1993). New developments in treating depression. *Audio-Digest, Psychiatry, 22*(07).

Sands, B. F. (1994). Medications for treatment of anxiety disorders. *Audio-Digest, Psychiatry, 23*(07).

Santor, D. A., Zuroff, D. C., Ramsay, J. O., Cervantes, P., & Palacios, J. (1994). Examining scale discriminability in the BDI and CES-D as a function of depressive severity. *Psychological Assessment, 7*, 131–139.

Schildkraut, J. (1965). The catecholamine hypothesis of affective disorders: A review of supporting evidence. *American Journal of Psychiatry, 122*, 509–522.

Schmaling, K., & Becker, J. (1991). Empirical studies of the interpersonal relations of adult depressives. In J. Becker & A. Kleinman (Eds.), *Psychosocial aspects of depression* (pp. 169–185). Hillsdale, NJ: Erlbaum.

Schulman, E. A. (1995). Current management of migraine. *Audio-Digest, Psychiatry, 24*(12).

Schulte, C. A. (1993). New classification of HIV infection. *Audio-Digest, Psychiatry, 22* (14).

Schwab, J. J. (1993). Combining psychotherapy and psychopharmacology in the treatment of depression in the family. *Audio-Digest, Psychiatry, 22* (17).

Schwartz, R. B., Komaroff, A. L., Garada, B. M., Gleit, M., Doolittle, T. H., Bates, D. W., Vasile, R. G., & Holman, B. L. (1994). SPECT imaging of the brain: Comparison of findings in patients with chronic fatigue syndrome,

AIDS dementia complex, and major unipolar depression. *ALR American Journal of Roentgenology, 162,* 943.

Scogin, F., Hamblin, D., & Seutler, L. (1987). Bibliotherapy for depressed older adults: A self-help alternative. *Gerontologist, 27*(3), 383–387.

Scogin, F., Jamison, C., & Davis, N. (1990). Two-year follow-up of bibliotherapy for depression in older adults. *Journal of Consulting and Clinical Psychology, 58*(5), 665–667.

Scogin, F., Jamison, C., & Gochneaur, K. (1989). Comparative efficacy of cognitive and behavioral bibliotherapy for mildly and moderately depressed older adults. *Journal of Consulting and Clinical Psychology, 57,* 403–407.

Scott, M., & Stadling, S. (1990). Group cognitive therapy for depression produces clinically significant reliable change in community-based settings. *Behavioral Psychotherapy, 18,* 1–19.

Seligman, M. E. P. (1975). *Helplessness: On depression, development, and death.* San Francisco: W.H. Freeman.

Seligman, M. E. P., & Maier, S. F. (1967). Failure to escape traumatic shock. *Journal of Experimental Psychology, 74,* 1–9.

Settle, Edmund C., Jr. (1993). Side effects of antidepressants. *Audio-Digest, Psychiatry, 22*(18).

Shaffer, D. (1988). The epidemiology of teen suicide: An examination of risk factors. *Journal of Clinical Psychiatry, 9* (Suppl.), 36–41.

Shapiro, R. W., Block, E., Rafaelson, O. J., Ryder, L. P., & Svejgaard, A. (1976). Histocompatibility antigens and manic depressive disorders. *Archives of General Psychiatry, 33,* 823–825.

Shaw, B., & Olmstead, M. (1989). *Competency ratings in relation to protocol adherence and clinical outcome.* Paper presented at the Society for Psychotherapy Research, Toronto, Canada.

Shea, M., Glass, D., Pilkonis, P., Watkins, J., & Docherty, J. (1987). Frequency and implications of personality disorders in a sample of depressed outpatients. *Journal of Personality Disorders, 1,* 27–42.

Sherbourne, C., Hays, R., Ordway, L., DiMatteo, M., & Kravitz, R. L. (1992). Antecedents of adherence to medical recommendations: Results from the medical outcomes study. *Journal of Behavioral Medicine, 15*(5), 447–468.

Shore, K. (1995). Managed care as a totalitarian regime. *The Independent Practitioner, 15*(2), 73–76.

Shure, D. M., Campes, F. E., & Eccleston, E. G. (1967). 5-hydroxytryptamine in the hind brain of depressive suicides. *British Journal of Psychiatry, 113,* 1407–1411.

Siever, L. J., & Davis, K. L. (1985). Overview: Toward a dysregulation hypothesis of depression. *American Journal of Psychiatry, 142,* 1017–1031.

Sifneos, P. E. (1973). The prevalence of "alexithymic" characteristics in psychosomatic patients. *Psychotherapy and Psychosomatios, 22,* 255–262.

Sifneos, P. E. (1979). *Short-term dynamic psychotherapy: Evaluation and technique.* New York: Plenum Press.

Silverman, W. H., & Beech, R. P. (1979). Are dropouts, dropouts? *Journal of Community Psychology, 7,* 236–242.

Silvestri, R., Montagnese, C., de Domenico, P., Raffaele, M., Casella, C., Lombardo, N., & Di-Perri, R. (1991). Narcolepsy and psychopathology: A case report. *Acta Neurologica, 13*(3), 275–278.

Sims, A. (1977). Prognosis in the neurosis. *American Journal of Psychoanalysis, 37,* 155–161.

Sluijs, E., & Knibbe, J. (1991). Patient compliance with exercise: Different theoretical approaches to short-term and long-term compliance. *Patient Education & Counseling, 17*(3), 191–204.

Smith, D., & Burkhalter, J. (1987). The use of bibliotherapy in clinical practice. *Journal of Mental Health Counseling, 9*(3), 184–190.

Smith, K. M., Merritt, S. L., & Cohen, F. L. (1992). Can we predict cognitive impairments in persons with narcolepsy? *Loss, Grief & Care, 5*(3-4), 103–113.

Smucker, M. R., & Craighead, W. E. (1986). Normative and reliability data for the Children's depression inventory. *Journal of Abnormal Child Psychology, 14*(1), 25–39.

Smuts, J. C. (1961). *Holism and evolution.* New York: Viking.

Snaith, P. (1993). What do depression rating scales measure? *British Journal of Psychiatry, 163,* 293–298.

Snaith, R. P., Ahmed, S. N., Mehta, S., & Hamilton, M. (1971). Assessment of the severity of primary depressive illness: Wakefield self-assessment depression inventory. *Psychological Medicine, 1,* 143–149.

Solomon, D. A., Keitner, G. I., Miller, I. W., Shea, M. T., & Keller, M. B. (1995). Course of illness and maintenance treatments for patients with bipolar disorder. *Journal of Clinical Psychiatry, 56*(1), 5–13.

Spaner, D., Bland, R., & Newman, S. (1994). Major depressive disorder. *Acta Psychiatrica Scandinavica, 89*(376, Suppl.), 7–15.

Sperry, L., & Carlson, J. (1993). *Psychopathology and psychotherapy: From diagnosis to treatment.* Muncie, IN: Accelerated Development.

Spevak, P. (1982). A multi-strategy approach to the maintenance of personal fitness programs. *Dissertation Abstracts International, 42*(8–B), 3445, University of Missouri, Columbia.

Spevak, P., & Richards, C. (1980). Enhancing the durability of treatment effects: Maintenance strategies in the treatment of nail-biting. *Cognitive Therapy & Research, 4*(2), 251–258.

Spilker, B. (1992). Methods of assessing and improving patient compliance in clinical trials. *IRB: A Review of Human Subjects Research, 14*(3), 1–6.

Spitzer, R. L., Endicott, J., & Robins, E. (1978). Research diagnostic criteria: Rationale and reliability. *Archives of General Psychiatry, 35,* 773–782.

Spoerl, O. H. (1975). Single session-psychotherapy (Abstract). *Diseases of the Nervous System, 36,* 283–285.

Stark, K. D. (1990). *Childhood depression: School-based intervention.* New York: Guilford Press.

References 227

Starker, S. (1988). Do-it-yourself therapy: The prescription of self-help books by psychologists. *Psychotherapy, 25,* 142–146.

St. Dennis, C. (1995, June 29). *New advances in the treatment of depression: Emphasizing the serotonin receptor.* Talk given at Sacred Heart Medical Center, Providence Auditorium, Spokane, WA.

Stein, P. N., & Motta, R. W. (1992). Effects of aerobic and nonaerobic exercise on depression and self-concept. *Perceptual & Motor Skills, 74*(1), 79–89.

Stich, T. F., & Senior, N. (1984) Adventure therapy: An innovative treatment for psychiatric patients. *New Directions for Mental Health Services, 21,* 103–108.

Stone, A. A. (1995). Psychotherapy and managed care: The bigger picture. *The Harvard Mental Health Letter, 11*(8), 5–7.

Stone, L. (1986). Psychoanalytic observations on the pathology of depressive illness: Selected spheres of ambiguity and disagreement. *Journal of the American Psychoanalytic Association, 34,* 329–362.

Stoudemire, A., Frank, R., Hedemark, N., Kamlet, M., & Blazer, D. (1986). The economic burden of depression. *General Hospital Psychiatry, 8,* 387–394.

Strauss, C. C., Last, C. G., Hersen, M., & Kuzdin, A. E. (1988). Association between anxiety and depression in children and adolescents with anxiety disorders. *Journal of Abnormal Child Psychology, 16,* 57–68.

Strober, M. (1984). Familial aspects of depressive disorder in early adolescence. In E. Weller & R. Weller (Eds.), *Current perspectives on major depressive disorders in children* (pp. 38–48). Washington, DC: American Psychiatric Press.

Strober, M., Hanna, G., & McCracken, J. (1989). Bipolar disorder. In C. G. Last & M. Hersen (Eds.), *Handbook of child psychiatric diagnosis* (pp. 299–316). New York: Wiley.

Strober, M., & Katz, J. L. (1987). Depression in the eating disorders: A review and analysis of descriptive, family, and biological findings. In D. Garner & P. Garfinkel (Eds.), *Diagnostic issues in eating disorders* (pp. 80–111). New York: Brunner/Mazel.

Strober, M., Morrell, W., Lampert, C., & Burroughs, J. (1990). Relapse following discontinuation of lithium maintenance therapy in adolescents with bipolar I illness: A naturalistic study. *American Journal of Psychiatry, 147,* 457–461.

Strupp, H. H. (1992). The future of psychodynamic psychotherapy. *Psychotherapy, 29*(1), 21.

Strupp. H. H., & Binder, J. L. (1984). *Psychotherapy in a new key: A guide to time-limited dynamic psychotherapy.* New York: Basic Books.

Stunkard, A. J., & Rush, J. (1974). Dieting and depression reexamined. *Annals of Internal Medicine, 81,* 526–533.

Sturm, R., Jackson, C. A., Meredith, L. S., Yip, W., Manning, W. G., Rogers, W. H., & Wells, K. B. (1995). Mental health care utilization in prepaid and fee-for-service plans among depressed patients in the Medical Outcomes Study. *Health Services Research, 30*(2), 319–340.

Sturm, R., & Wells, K. B. (1995). How can care for depression become more cost-effective? *Journal of the American Medical Association, 273*(1), 51–58.

Sundram, C. J., & Johnson, P. W. (1992). The legal aspects of narcolepsy. *Loss, Grief & Care, 5*(3–4), 175–192.

Swinson, R. (1994). *Panic disorder, social phobia and depression: The clinical interface.* Mississauga, Ontario: Canadian Psychiatric Association.

Talley, J. E. (1992). *The predictors of successful very brief psychotherapy: A study of differences by gender, age, and treatment variables.* Springfield, IL: Thomas.

Talley, J. H. (1994). Anxiety and depression. *Audio-Digest, Family Practice, 42*(04).

Talmon, M. (1990). *Single-session brief therapy.* San Francisco: Jossey-Bass.

Tangney, J. P. (1993). Shame and guilt. In C. G. Costello (Ed.), *Symptoms of depression* (pp. 161–180). New York: Wiley.

Tannenbaum, L., & Forehand, R. (1994). Maternal depressive mood: The role of the father in preventing adolescent problem behaviors. *Behavior Research & Therapy, 32*(3), 321–325.

Targum, S. D., Dibble, E. D., Davenport, Y. B., & Gershon, E. S. (1981). Family attitudes questionnaire: Patients and spouses view bipolar illness. *Archives of General Psychiatry, 38,* 562–568.

Teri, L., & Lewinsohn, P. (1986). Individual and group treatment of unipolar depression: Comparison of treatment outcome and identification of predictors of successful treatment outcome. *Behavior Therapy, 17,* 215–228.

Terman, M., Botticelli, S., Link, B., Link, M., Hardin, T., & Rosenthal, N. (1989). Seasonal symptom patterns in New York: Patients and population. In T. Silverton & C. Thompson (Eds.), *Seasonal affective disorder* (pp. 77–95). London: Clinical Neuroscience Publishers.

Terman, M., Williams, J., & Terman, J. (1991). Light therapy for winter depression: A clinician's guide. In P. Keller (Ed.), *Innovations in clinical practice: A source book* (pp. 179–221). Sarasota, FL: Pro Resource.

Thase, M. E. (1994). Cognitive-behavioral therapy of severe unipolar depression. In L. Grunhaus & J. F. Greden (Eds.), *Severe depressive disorders* (pp. 269–296). Washington, DC: American Psychiatric Press.

Thompson, L., Gallagher, D., & Breckenridge, J. (1987). Comparative effectiveness of psychotherapies for depressed elders. *Journal of Consulting and Clinical Psychology, 55*(3), 385–390.

Tiller, J. W. G. (1990). Antidepressants, alcohol, and psychomotor performance. *Acta Psychiatrica Scandinavica, 360*(Suppl.), 13–17.

Toennies, F. (1940). *(Gemeinschaft und Gesellschaft) Fundamental concepts of sociology.* (C. P. Loomis, Trans.). New York: American Book.

Trick, L. (1993). Patient compliance: Don't count on it! *Journal of the American Optometric Association, 64*(4), 264–270.

Trimble, M. (1995). Anticonvulsants. *Audio-Digest, Psychiatry, 24*(07).

Tulkin, S., Frank, G., Bernstein, A., Aubel, B., & Lehn, M. (1992). Management of chronic benign pain in a prepaid practice. In J. Feldman & R. Fitzpatrick (Eds.), *Managed mental health care: Administrative and clinical issues.* Washington, DC: American Psychiatric Press.

Turnbull, J. M. (1994). Anxiety and physical illness in the elderly. *Audio-Digest, Internal Medicine, 42*(01).

Turner, J. A., & Denny, M. C. (1993). Do antidepressant medications relieve chronic low back pain? *Journal of Family Practice, 37*(6), 545–553.

Tyler, S., & Brittlebank, A. (1993). Misdiagnosis of bipolar affective disorder as personality disorder. *Canadian Journal of Psychiatry, 38*(9), 587–589.

Uars, X., & Hoyt, M. (1992). The managed care movement and the future of psychotherapy. *Psychotherapy, 29*(1), 109–118.

Udry, E. M. (1992). Interventions for the anxious and depressed: Suggested links between control theory and exercise therapy. *Journal of Reality Therapy, 12*(1), 32–36.

Van Egmond, M., & Diekstra, R. F. W. (1989). The predictability of suicidal behavior. In R. F. W. Diekstra, R. Maris, & S. Platt (Eds.), *The role of attitude and imitations.* Leiden, Netherlands: E. J. Brill.

VandenBos, G. R., DeLeon, P. H., & Belar, C. D. (1991). How many psychological practitioners are needed? It's too early to know. *Professional Psychology: Research and Practice, 22*(6), 441–448.

Vaughn, C. E., & Leff, J. P. (1976). The measurement of expressed emotion in the families of psychiatric patients. *British Journal of Social and Clinical Psychology, 15*, 157–165.

Veith, R. C., Raskind, M. A., Caldwell, J. H., Barnes, R. F., Gumbrecht, G., & Ritchie, J. L. (1982). Cardiovascular effects of the tricyclic antidepressants in depressed patients with chronic heart disease. *New England Journal of Medicine, 306*, 954–955.

Verhulst, J. (1995, March). *The medical and the narrative method in psychiatry.* Talk given at Ground Rounds, Department of Psychiatry, University of Washington, Seattle.

Volkan, V. D. (1994). *Depressive states and their treatment.* Northvale, NJ: Jason Aronson.

von Bertalanffy, L. (1968). *General systems theory.* New York: Braziller.

Von Knorring, A., Cloninger, C. R., Bohman, M., & Sigvardsson, A. (1983). An adoption study of depressive disorders and substance abuse. *Archives of General Psychiatry, 40*, 943–950.

von Korff, M., Ormel, J., Katon, W., & Lin, E. (1992). Disability and depression among high utilizers of health care: A longitudinal analysis. *Archives of General Psychiatry, 49*, 91–100.

Walker, E., Katon, A., Harrop-Griffiths, J., Holm, L., Russo, J., & Hickok, L. (1988). Relationship of chronic pelvic pain to psychiatric diagnoses and childhood sexual abuse. *American Journal of Psychiatry, 145*(1), 75–80.

Walker, L. S., & Greene, J. W. (1989). Children with recurrent abdominal pain and their parents: More somatic complaints, anxiety, and depression than other patient families. *Journal of Pediatric Psychology, 14*(2), 231–243.

Walter, J. L., & Peller, J. E. (1992). *Becoming solution-focused in brief therapy.* New York: Brunner/Mazel.

Wamboidt, M. Z. (1993). Pediatric medical and psychiatric comorbidity. *Audio-Digest, Psychiatry, 22*(19).

Waring, E., Patton, D., & Wister, A. (1990). The etiology of nine psychotic emotional illnesses. *Canadian Journal of Psychiatry, 35*(1), 50–57.

Warner, R. (1991). Bibliotherapy: A comparison of the prescription practices of Canadian and American psychologists. *Canadian Psychology, 32*(3), 529–530.

Wegner, G. (1993). The information of social networks: Self-help, mutual aid, and old people in contemporary Britain. *Journal of Aging Studies, 7*(1), 25–40.

Wehr, T. A., & Goodwin, F. K. (1987). Do antidepressants cause mania? *Psychopharmacology Bulletin, 23*, 61–65.

Weissman, M. M. (1979). The psychological treatment of depression: Evidence for the efficacy of psychotherapy alone, and in comparison with, and in combination with pharmacotherapy. *Archives of General Psychiatry, 36*, 1261–1269.

Weissman, M. M., Klerman, G. L., Prusoff, B. A., Sholomskas, D., & Padian, N. (1981). Depressed outpatients: Results one year after treatment with drugs and/or interpersonal psychotherapy. *Archives of General Psychiatry, 36*, 51–55.

Weissman, M. M., & Myers, J. (1978). Affective disorders in a U.S. urban community: The use of Research Diagnostic Criteria in an epidemiologic study. *Archives of General Psychiatry, 35*, 1304–1311.

Weissman, M., & Myers, J. (1980). Psychiatric disorders in a U.S. urban community: The application of Research Diagnostic Criteria to a re-surveyed community sample. *Acta Psychiatrica Scandinavica, 62*, 99–111.

Weissman, M. M., Prusoff, B., & Newberry, P. B. (1975). *Comparison of CES-D, Zung, Beck self-report depression scales* (Technical Report ADM 42-47-83). Rockville, MD: Center for Epidemiologic Studies, National Institute of Mental Health.

Weitzler, K., Strauman, J., & Dubro, A. (1989). Diagnosis of major depression by self-report. *Journal of Personality Assessment, 53*(1), 22–30.

Weller, E., & Weller, R. (1990). Depressive disorders in children and adolescents. In B. Garfinkel, G. Carlson, & E. Weller (Eds.), *Psychiatric disorders in children and adolescents* (pp. 3–20). Philadelphia: W. B. Saunders.

Wells, K. B. (1985). *Depression as a tracer condition for the national study of medical care outcomes—background review.* Santa Monica, CA: RAND.

Wells, K. B., Astrachan, B. M., Tischler, G. L., & Unutzer, J. (1995). Issues and approaches in evaulating managed mental health care. *Milbank Quarterly, 73*(1), 57–75.

Wells, K. B., Burnam, M. A., & Camp, P. (1995). Severity of depression in prepaid and fee-for-service general medical and mental health specialty practices. *Medical Care, 33*(4), 350–364.

Wells, K. B., Golding, J. M., & Burnam, M. A. (1988). Psychiatric disorder and limitations in physical functioning in a sample of the Los Angeles general population. *American Journal of Psychiatry, 145*, 712–717.

Wells, K. B., Stewart, A., Hays, R., Burnam, M., Rogers, W., Daniels, M., Berry, S., Greenfeld, S., & Ware, J. (1989). The functioning and well-being of depressed patients: Results from the Medical Outcomes Study. *Journal of the American Medical Association, 262*(7), 914–919.

Wesner, R. B., & Winokur, G. (1990). Genetics of affective disorders. In B. B.

Wolman & G. Stricker (Eds.), *Depressive disorders: Facts, theories, and treatment methods* (pp. 125–146). New York: Wiley.

Wiggins, J. G. (1994). Is psychology relevant to managed care?: Some implications for state health care reform. *Psychotherapy Bulletin, 29*(4), 30–31.

Wilcox, J. (1986). Psychopathology and narcolepsy. *Neuropsychobiology,* 14(4), 170–172.

Willenbring, M. (1986). Measurement of depression in alcoholics. *Journal of Studies of Alcohol, 47*(5), 367–372.

Williams, J. M. G. (1992). *The psychological treatment of depression: A guide to the theory and practice of cognitive behavior therapy* (2nd ed.). New York: Routledge.

Williamson, D., Birmaher, B., Anderson, B., Al-Shabbout, M., & Ryan, N. (1995). Stressful life events in depressed adolescents: The role of dependent events during the depressive episode. *Journal of the American Academy of Child & Adolescent Psychiatry, 34*(5), 591–598.

Williamson, G. M., & Schulz, R. (1992). Physical illness and symptoms of depression among elderly outpatients. *Psychology and Aging, 7,* 343–351.

Willner, P. (1993). Anhedonia. In C. G. Costello (Ed.), *Symptoms of depression* (pp. 63–84). New York: Wiley.

Wing, J. K, Birley, J., Cooper, J., Graham, P., & Isaacs, A. (1967). Reliability of a procedure for measuring and classifying "Present Psychiatric State." *British Journal of Psychiatry, 113,* 499–515.

Wing, J. K., Mann, S. A., Leff, J. P., & Nixon, J. M. (1978). The concept of a "case" in psychiatric population surveys. *Psychological Medicine, 8,* 203–217.

Winstead, D. (1994). Resperidone and clozapine. *Audio-Digest, Psychiatry, 23*(10).

Wolbert, L. (1967). *Short-term psychotherapy.* New York: Grune & Stratton.

Wollersheim, J., & Wilson, G. (1991). Group treatment of unipolar depression: A comparison of coping, supportive, bibliotherapy, and delayed treatment groups. *Professional Psychology: Research and Practice, 22*(6), 496–502.

Wolman, B. B., & Stricker, G. (1990). *Depressive disorders: Facts, theories, and treatment methods.* New York: Wiley.

Wolpe, J. (1972). Neurotic depression: Experimental analog, clinical syndromes and treatment. *American Journal of Psychotherapy, 25,* 362–368.

Woody, J. (1990). Clinical strategies to promote compliance. *American Journal of Family Therapy, 18*(3), 285–294.

Woolhander, S., & Himmelstein, D. U. (1991). The deteriorating administrative effeciency of the U.S. health care system. *New England Journal of Medicine, 324,* 1253–1258.

Wu, J. C., Gillin, J. L., Buchsbaum, M. S., Hershey, T., Johnson, J. L., & Bunney, W. E., Jr. (1992). Effect of sleep deprivation on brain metabolism of depressed patients. *American Journal of Psychiatry, 149,* 538.

Young, J. (1989). Schema-focussed cognitive therapy for difficult patients and characterological disorders. Workshop presented at World Congress of Cognitive Therapy, Oxford, England.

Youssel, F. (1983). Compliance with therapeutic regimens: A follow-up study for patients with affective disorders. *Journal of Advance Nursing, 8,* 513–517.

Zapotocsky, H. (1992). Psychotherapy of depression. 7th Psychiatric Forum:

Actual aspects of depression (1991, Salzburg, Austria). *Psychiatria Danubina,* *4*(1–2), 141–143.

Zavodnick, S. (1990). Somatic therapies of depression. In B. B. Wolman & G. Sticker (Eds.), *Depressive disorders: Facts, theories, and treatment methods* (pp. 275–295). New York: Wiley.

Ziegler, V. E., Co, B. T., Taylor, D. R., Clayton, P. J., & Biggs, J. T. (1976). Amitriptyline plasma levels and therapeutic response. *Clinical Pharmacology and Therapeutics, 19,* 795–801.

Zimbardo, P. G. (1977). *Shyness: What it is, what to do about it.* Reading, MA: Addison-Wesley.

Zimet, C. N. (1979). Developmental task and crisis groups. *Psychotherapy, 16,* 2–8.

Zisook, S., & Shuchter, S. (1991). Depression through the first year after the death of a spouse. *American Journal of Psychiatry, 148*(10), 1346–1352.

Zoega, T., Barr, C., & Barsky, A. (1991). Prediction of compliance with medication and follow-up appointments. *Nordisk Psykiatrisk Tidsskrift, 45*(1), 27–32.

Zung, W. (1969). A cross-cultural survey of symptoms in depression. *American Journal of Psychiatry, 126*(1), 116–121.

Zung, W. W. K. (1965). A self-rating depression scale. *Archives of General Psychiatry, 12,* 63–70.

Name Index

Subject Index